Empowering Pain Management

A Comprehensive Practical Guide to Mastering Life with Chronic Pain

Dr Arul James
MBBS MD FRCA FFPMRCA

Consultant Chronic Pain Medicine

Contents

How to Use This Book to Manage Chronic Pain

This book offers abundant knowledge regarding diverse elements of managing chronic pain. To maximise the benefits of this guide, I have provided some practical tips in this chapter for successfully utilising this book in your chronic pain management journey.

STEP ONE: START WITH THE BASICS

Begin by reading the first few chapters, which will give you a fundamental understanding and enhance your comprehension of the mechanisms of pain and the diverse methods of handling it.

Chapter 1. Science of Pain
Chapter 2. Personalised Pain Management Plan
Chapter 3. Alternative and Complementary Therapies

STEP TWO: FIND YOUR GOALS

Take time to reflect on your pain management goals. What are your top priorities? Do you want to reduce pain intensity, improve function, or enhance your quality of life?

Chapter 4. Finding Balance

STEP THREE: EXPLORE DIFFERENT TREATMENT APPROACHES

This book covers a range of treatment approaches. Please read about the strategies that interest you. By being informed and proactive in your pain management, you can certainly take control of your life and work towards living it to the fullest.

Chapter 5. Mind-Body Techniques
Chapter 6. Managing Chronic Pain Through Meditation
Chapter 7. Yoga for Chronic Pain
Chapter 8. Tai Chi for Managing Chronic Pain
Chapter 9. Nutrition and Chronic Pain
Chapter 10. Transcutaneous Electrical Nerve Stimulation
Chapter 11. Cognitive Behavioural Therapy (CBT)
Chapter 12. Specialised Care for Chronic Pain

STEP FOUR: EXPERIMENT WITH COPING STRATEGIES

Managing chronic pain requires a combination of medical interventions and coping strategies. These chapters offer practical tips for managing pain in daily life. Try out different methods and find which ones work best for you.

Chapter 13. Coping with Flares and Exacerbations
Chapter 14. Sleep Management for Chronic Pain
Chapter 15. Mood and Chronic Pain
Chapter 16. Effective Activity Pacing
Chapter 17. Somatic Exercises to Ease Chronic Pain

STEP FIVE: BUILD A SUPPORT SYSTEM

Managing chronic pain can be challenging, but you don't have to do it alone. This book offers further chapters that guide you to build a support system and navigate relationships.

Chapter 18. Building a Support System

Remember, chronic pain management is an ongoing process that may require experimentation and testing to find what works best for you.

Preface

Chronic pain affects millions of individuals worldwide, significantly impacting their overall quality of life. In this book, I aim to provide practical guidance and comprehensive solutions to help you conquer chronic pain.

I have compiled a wealth of information on various aspects of chronic pain management. This book will undoubtedly be a valuable tool not just for those living with chronic pain but also for healthcare professionals, family members and friends who provide support and care to those living with chronic pain.

Together, we can work towards creating a world where individuals with chronic pain have access to the resources and support needed to better manage their chronic pain and, in turn, maximise their quality of life.

Step One: Start With the Basics

1. Science of Pain

Understanding the Physiology and Psychology of Chronic Pain

INTRODUCTION

Chronic pain is a significant health concern which has profound impact on millions of people worldwide. It has the potential to cause physical, emotional, and psychological distress, which can negatively affect a person's quality of life. It's crucial to recognise that pain encompasses not only physical sensations but also psychological and emotional aspects. This chapter will explore the science behind chronic pain, including its physiology and psychology, to help you better understand what happens in your body and mind when you experience chronic pain. In addition, we will discuss the different types of chronic pain and the various factors that can cause or worsen chronic pain.

IMPORTANCE OF UNDERSTANDING THE PHYSIOLOGY AND PSYCHOLOGY OF PAIN

Understanding the science of chronic pain is crucial for effective pain management. It can help you make knowledgeable choices about the most suitable treatments for your condition, such as medicines, physiotherapy, and complementary therapies. Additionally, understanding the psychology of pain can help you develop coping strategies to manage your pain and improve your quality of life. It is crucial to bear in mind that chronic pain is a complex condition capable of affecting every aspect of your life. However, it is possible to manage chronic pain and regain control over your life with the proper support, knowledge, and tools.

WHAT IS PAIN?

Pain is an unpleasant sensation initiated by the nervous system when it senses potential or actual tissue damage. Pain is like a warning signal that tells us something is wrong and prompts us to protect ourselves from further harm.

ANALOGY

Imagine pain as a warning signal. Just like a smoke detector warns you when there's a fire, pain is your body's way of telling you something is wrong. It's a signal to act and protect yourself from further harm.

DISTINGUISHING SHORT-TERM (ACUTE) PAIN AND LONG-TERM (CHRONIC) PAIN

Acute pain is a natural response to tissue damage which typically resolves within a few days or weeks. Chronic pain is when you have pain for more than three months and needs a different way of taking care of it than short-term pain.

ANALOGY

Think of your body's alarm system like a car alarm. Just like a car alarm goes off when there's a potential threat, such as a break-in, your body's alarm system triggers when it senses danger, such as an injury or inflammation. However, in persistent pain, this alarm system can become overly sensitive and start going off even when there's no real danger. It's like a car alarm that goes off whenever a leaf falls on the car instead of only when someone tries to break in. In chronic pain, the alarm system is constantly sounding the alarm, even though there may not be any actual harm occurring. This is why managing chronic pain requires a different approach than managing acute pain.

PHYSIOLOGY OF PAIN

When tissue damage occurs, specialised cells called nociceptors are activated. They send signals to the spinal cord, which then relays these signals to the brain, where they are processed and interpreted as pain. The brain then generates a pain experience, which can include a range of sensory, emotional, and cognitive components.

The release of chemicals in response to tissue damage also plays a role in the physiology of pain. For example, inflammatory chemicals can sensitise nociceptors, making them more responsive to pain signals. Other chemicals, such as endorphins, can reduce pain signals and produce feelings of euphoria or well-being.

In addition to nociceptors, there are other types of nerve cells that play a role in the physiology of pain. For example, there are nerve cells that send information about the location and intensity of the pain, as well as nerve cells that modulate pain signals and can either amplify or reduce the pain experience.

Pain is transmitted through the nervous system, which means that pain signals can be amplified or dampened depending on the state of your nervous system. This is why stress, anxiety, and other emotional factors can worsen pain symptoms.

ANALOGY

An analogy for the nervous system's role in amplifying or dampening pain signals could be comparing it to the volume control on a stereo system. Just like how turning up the volume makes the music louder, the state of your nervous system can amplify pain signals and make them feel more intense. On the other hand, just as turning down the volume makes music quieter, reducing stress and anxiety can dampen pain signals and make them feel less intense. By understanding the role of the nervous system and how it interacts with emotional factors, you can learn how to enhance your pain management skills and minimise its impact on your daily life.

PSYCHOLOGY OF PAIN

Pain is more than just a physical sensation; it also involves psychological and emotional factors. For example, anxiety, depression, and stress can all worsen pain symptoms. This is partly because these conditions can activate the sympathetic nervous system, which can increase your sensitivity to pain.

In addition, pain can cause changes in the brain that lead to a heightened sensitivity to pain. This occurs because chronic pain has the potential to induce a phenomenon referred to as central sensitisation, where the nervous system becomes hyperactive and more responsive to pain signals. This can make pain harder to deal with and cause other symptoms like tiredness, trouble sleeping, and feeling down.

The psychology of pain also includes the way that pain is perceived and interpreted by the individual. For example, two people with the same type and severity of pain may have quite different experiences of pain, depending on their beliefs, expectations, and past experiences with pain. This means that pain management approaches that consider the individual's psychological and emotional factors can be highly effective in managing chronic pain.

TYPES OF CHRONIC PAIN

Chronic pain can occur secondary to various factors, including injury, disease, or inflammation. Injuries, such as those resulting from accidents or trauma, can damage tissues in the body and lead to chronic pain. Conditions like arthritis or fibromyalgia can also cause chronic pain by affecting the joints, muscles, or nerves. Inflammation, a natural response of the body to injury or infection, can cause pain that persists long after the initial injury or disease has resolved. Chronic pain can be classified into different types; neuropathic pain arises from the impairment or malfunctioning of the nerves, while musculoskeletal pain is caused by issues with muscles, bones, or joints. Other types of chronic pain include visceral pain, which originates from internal organs, or headaches, which can have various triggers and underlying mechanisms.

CONCLUSION

Understanding the science of pain can help you better manage your chronic pain symptoms. By learning about the physiology and psychology of pain, you can better understand what's happening in your body and mind when you experience pain. This can help you make well-informed decisions about your treatment choices and take necessary measures to manage your pain more efficiently.

2. Personalised Pain Management Plan

Understanding the importance of personalising
your pain management strategy

INTRODUCTION

There is no universal solution for dealing with chronic pain management. Every person's encounter with persistent pain is distinctive, and strategies that are effective for one individual may not be for someone else. That's why it's essential to personalise your pain management plan and explore different approaches to find what works best for you. This chapter will discuss the importance of creating a personalised pain management plan and explore various approaches to managing chronic pain, including medication, physical therapy, alternative therapies, and psychological techniques.

ANALOGIES

Here are some analogies for the importance of personalising your pain management plan:

Pain management is like gardening. Every plant needs a different type of soil, sunlight, and water to thrive. Similarly, every patient requires different therapies to manage their pain successfully.

Personalising your pain management plan is like solving a puzzle. Each person's experience with chronic pain is different. Therefore, the best pain management plan will require fitting together various pieces to create a unique solution that works for each person.

TRYING DIFFERENT APPROACHES TO PAIN MANAGEMENT

Exploring different approaches to pain management is crucial because there is no single solution to managing chronic pain. Different therapies and treatments may work better for different people. Finding what works for you may require some time and trial and error. Combining various therapies can more effectively manage chronic pain than relying on a single approach. That's why it's essential to try different approaches to pain management. By exploring different methods, you can find what works best for you and create a comprehensive pain management plan that includes a combination of therapies.

One commonly used method is taking medication, including over-the-counter pain relievers, prescription painkillers, and other drugs. However, medication is not always the most effective option, and it can come with risks and side effects.

Physical therapy is an option that can be very helpful for some people with chronic pain. One way to manage pain and improve physical function is through exercise and other techniques that aim to enhance strength, flexibility, and range of motion while alleviating pain.

Cognitive-behavioural therapy (CBT) is a type of talk therapy which can be helpful in managing chronic pain. This approach emphasises modifying negative thoughts and behaviours that may worsen pain while teaching coping strategies and relaxation methods.

In addition to these traditional approaches, alternative therapies such as acupuncture, massage, and meditation may also be helpful for some people with chronic pain. These approaches can help decrease your stress and promote relaxation, which can, in turn, help alleviate your pain.

In general, it's important to be open-minded and willing to try various methods until you find the one that suits you best.

PERSONALISED TREATMENT PLAN

A personalised treatment plan is essential because it considers your unique needs and goals. Tailor your pain management plan; it involves collaborating closely with your healthcare professionals to design a treatment plan that considers your specific requirements. Your medical practitioner will evaluate your pain and identify any underlying conditions that could be causing it. They will also consider your medical history, lifestyle factors, and any other treatments or medications you may be taking.

Using the information gathered, your healthcare provider will create a customised treatment strategy that meets your unique requirements. This may include a combination of different therapies, such as medications, physical therapy, behavioural therapy, or alternative treatments like acupuncture or massage therapy. Your healthcare team will discuss with you to create a plan that considers your pain levels, lifestyle, and medical history. Your provider will also work with you to set realistic goals for pain relief and functional improvement.

It's important to remember that developing a personalised treatment plan is an ongoing process. Collaboration between you and your healthcare provider is necessary to monitor your progress and modify your treatment plan as necessary. Once you have a customised treatment plan, you can be assured that you are receiving the best care for your chronic pain.

CONCLUSION

In conclusion, managing chronic pain is a complex and continuous process that requires a personalised approach. Remember that managing chronic pain is a journey; it may take time to discover the most effective combination of treatments for your needs. However, by being patient, persistent, open to trying new things, and actively taking part in managing your pain, you have the power to enhance your overall well-being and take control of your life.

3. Alternative and Complementary Therapies

Exploring the Potential Benefits

INTRODUCTION

Chronic pain can be challenging to manage, and conventional medical treatments may not always provide adequate relief. As a result, many individuals are turning to alternative and complementary therapies in their search for pain relief. These therapies, which include TENS, acupuncture, chiropractic care, and other modalities, can provide a holistic approach to managing your pain and address both physical and emotional aspects of pain. This chapter will explore the potential benefits of these therapies and how they can help individuals manage chronic pain.

TENS

TENS therapy is a non-invasive treatment method that utilizes a low-level electrical current applied to the affected area to relieve pain. While it can be a helpful tool for some individuals in managing chronic pain, it may not be effective for everyone. The effectiveness of TENS therapy can also vary depending on the individual's pain condition and the severity of their symptoms.

ACUPUNCTURE

Acupuncture is an ancient practice which involves inserting fine needles into specific acupoints on the body to improve the circulation of Qi, or energy. There is some effectiveness of acupuncture in managing various chronic pain conditions, including lower back pain, osteoarthritis, and migraine headaches. While acupuncture is effective for certain conditions, the exact mechanism of action is not fully comprehended; it is believed that the treatment functions by stimulating the body's natural anti-inflammatory and pain-relieving processes.

CHIROPRACTIC CARE

Chiropractic care provides a drug-free and non-invasive method of managing chronic pain that can offer some effectiveness in managing chronic pain, including back and neck pain. Chiropractors use spinal manipulation, massage, and other techniques to enhance spinal alignment and relieve pressure on the nervous system. Chiropractors may also use other modalities, such as ultrasound and electrical stimulation, to enhance the effectiveness of treatment.

MASSAGE THERAPY

Massage therapy is a technique that involves manipulating soft tissues within the body to help with relaxation, improve circulation, and reduce pain and inflammation. Massage therapy has been found to provide some benefits in managing conditions such as fibromyalgia, osteoarthritis, and lower back pain. The benefits of massage therapy may be due to its ability to reduce muscle tension, increase the production of endorphins, and promote relaxation.

HEAT AND COLD THERAPY

The topical application of heat or cold to the affected region can aid in the reduction of pain and inflammation. Heat therapy, including the use of a heating pad or enjoying a warm bath, can relax muscles and improve circulation. Cold treatment, like an ice pack or a cold shower, can help numb the affected area and reduce swelling.

MIND-BODY THERAPIES

Mind-body therapies, which include meditation, yoga, and tai chi, have demonstrated effectiveness in managing chronic pain. These practices promote relaxation, reduce stress, and improve emotional well-being, which can help reduce pain perception. Mind-body therapies may also enhance the quality of sleep, which is vital for managing chronic pain.

CONCLUSION

Alternative and complementary therapies offer a non-invasive, drug-free approach to managing chronic pain. Although these therapies may not be effective for everyone, they are worth considering for individuals who have not found relief with conventional medical treatments. Consulting with a certified practitioner is advised to determine if it is a safe and appropriate treatment option for your individual needs. Combining alternative and complementary therapies, conventional medical treatments, and self-care strategies can improve your overall quality of life and manage the symptoms more effectively.

Step Two: Find Your Goals

4. Finding Balance

Setting Realistic Goals and Expectations for
a Fulfilling Life with Chronic Pain

INTRODUCTION

Living with chronic pain can present difficulties and be a burdensome experience. It can affect your physical, psychological, emotional, and social well-being, making it difficult to perform even the simplest tasks. But setting realistic goals and expectations can help you manage chronic pain and improve your quality of life. In this chapter, we will learn the significance of establishing achievable objectives and how to do it.

IMPORTANCE OF SETTING REALISTIC
GOALS AND EXPECTATIONS

Setting realistic goals and expectations is crucial for individuals with chronic pain as it can help break the cycle of pain and depression. When you set goals that are achievable and meaningful, it provides a sense of purpose and control over your life. It can also increase your motivation to engage in activities you enjoy, leading to a better quality of life.

On the other hand, setting unrealistic goals and expectations can lead to frustration and disappointment. This can cause you to feel helpless and discouraged, leading to increased pain and decreased quality of life.

Bear in mind that the experience of chronic pain is individual, so what is feasible for one person might not be for another. It's essential to focus on your abilities and limitations and be kind to yourself as you work towards your goals. Setting realistic goals and expectations allows you to take control of your life and increase your overall well-being.

ANALOGIES

Here are some analogies to help illustrate the concept of setting realistic goals and expectations.

- ○ *You can approach it similarly to how you would plan a journey or road trip - you wouldn't plan to drive from New York to California in one day, as it would be unrealistic and likely to leave you feeling overwhelmed and exhausted. Instead, you might plan to drive a certain number of miles each day, taking breaks and enjoying the journey.*

- ○ *Similarly, setting realistic goals and expectations for managing your chronic pain is like breaking the journey down into manageable steps. For example, consider setting a goal to walk for 10 minutes daily, gradually increasing the time as you become more comfortable. This way, you can feel a sense of accomplishment and progress each day rather than feeling discouraged and overwhelmed by an unattainable goal.*

- ○ *When setting goals, think of it like climbing a mountain. You don't start at the peak but rather take it step by step, resting when you need to and reassessing your progress. You may encounter setbacks, but that doesn't mean you can't keep moving forward.*

- ○ *Imagine you're running a race. You can't expect to start at the front of the pack if you haven't trained properly. Similarly, setting unrealistic goals for yourself can lead to disappointment and frustration. Instead, set achievable goals that will help you build momentum and improve your performance over time.*

- ○ *Just as it takes time and effort to grow a garden, it takes time and effort to achieve your goals. You have to prepare the soil, plant the seeds, water and tend to them regularly, and wait patiently for them to grow. Similarly, achieving your goals requires preparation, effort, and patience.*

○ *When building a house, you start with a solid foundation and work your way up. For example, you don't expect to move in right away but rather take the time to build each part of the house properly. Similarly, setting realistic goals means starting with a solid foundation, breaking down your larger goals into smaller, achievable steps, and building upon them over time.*

Remember, setting realistic goals and expectations is a process, not a destination. By taking small, manageable steps and focusing on progress rather than perfection, you can achieve your goals and improve your quality of life.

EASY STEPS TO SET YOUR GOALS

You can take the following steps to ensure you're heading in the right direction when establishing practical goals and expectations.

Step 1: Identify Your Desired Goal or Objective.

The first step involves recognising the desired outcome of treatment. This could be anything from spending time with loved ones to completing a task at work. It's important to choose goals that are meaningful to you and align with your values and priorities.

Step 2: Make Sure Your Goals Are Specific and Measurable.

Once you have identified your desired outcomes or goals, making them specific and measurable is essential. To illustrate, rather than setting a vague plan to increase physical activity, establish a clear and measurable goal, such as walking for 10 minutes three times a week. Doing so allows you to monitor your progress and acknowledge your accomplishments as you progress.

Step 3: Break Your Goals Down into Smaller Steps.

By dividing your goals into smaller, achievable tasks, you can maintain motivation and stay focused on your progress. For example, if your goal is to clean the house, break it down into smaller tasks, such as cleaning one room at a time.

Step 4: Be Realistic About Your Abilities.

It's important to be realistic about your abilities when setting goals. You may need to adjust your expectations based on your pain level or other limitations. For example, if you have chronic back pain, you may need to modify your exercise routine to avoid exacerbating your symptoms.

Step 5: Celebrate Your Achievements.

When you achieve a goal, no matter how small, take the time to celebrate your achievement. This will help to keep you motivated and focused on the progress you have made.

CONCLUSION

Setting realistic goals and expectations is a crucial part of managing chronic pain and improving your quality of life. By following the steps outlined in this chapter, you can set goals that are achievable, meaningful, and aligned with your values and priorities. It is important to practice self-compassion and patience towards oneself and to celebrate your achievements as you go through the process.

Step Three: Explore Different Treatment Approaches

5. Mind-Body Techniques

Harnessing the Power of Meditation, Yoga, and More
to Manage Pain and Enhance Well-Being

INTRODUCTION

Long-lasting pain can significantly affect an individual's daily functioning and quality of life, causing physical and emotional distress. While traditional medical treatments can be effective, the root cause of the pain may not always be effectively targeted by the treatment, provide relief from all symptoms, or have unwanted side effects. Mind-body techniques offer a holistic approach focusing on the link between a person's mental and physical states. They aim to promote relaxation, reduce stress and anxiety, and improve overall well-being. In this chapter, I will discuss how mind-body techniques can manage chronic pain and enhance well-being.

WHAT ARE MIND-BODY TECHNIQUES?

Mind-body techniques focus on the connection between the mind and body. These techniques can include meditation, yoga, tai chi, and other forms of relaxation and stress reduction. They are designed to help individuals achieve a state of relaxation, calmness, and focus, which can reduce stress and promote healing. These techniques are effective in managing chronic pain, which is often linked to stress and anxiety. When the body is under stress, it can worsen pain and inflammation, which can further increase stress and create a vicious cycle. Mind-body techniques can help break this cycle and improve well-being by reducing stress and promoting relaxation.

ANALOGY

Think of your mind and body as two separate instruments that need to work together in harmony. Similar to the way a musical instrument requires tuning and skilled playing to produce beautiful music, your mind and body need to be in balance to manage chronic pain effectively. Mind-body techniques can help you achieve this balance.

HOW CAN MIND-BODY TECHNIQUES HELP MANAGE CHRONIC PAIN?

Mind-body techniques are proven to be effective in managing chronic pain. They can help to reduce pain intensity, improve quality of life, and also decrease stress and anxiety. Mind-body techniques can also help you develop coping strategies to manage your pain more effectively.

ANALOGY

Think of the mind-body connection as a radio with two knobs - one for the mind and one for the body. Chronic pain can be like static interference, disrupting the signal between the mind and body. Mind-body techniques work by fine-tuning these knobs to improve the signal, leading to better pain management and overall well-being.

For example, meditation can help you develop a stronger mind-body connection. By focusing on the breath and quieting the mind, meditation can reduce stress and anxiety, which can often exacerbate pain. Similarly, yoga can help you improve flexibility, strengthen muscles, and reduce tension in the body. Tai chi is a type of therapy that emphasizes gentle movements and postures, which can also be effective in reducing pain and improving balance and coordination.

By incorporating mind-body techniques into your daily routine, you can actively manage your pain and improve your quality of life. These techniques provide a holistic approach to pain management, addressing both the physical and emotional aspects of pain. Just as tuning a radio requires patience and practice, incorporating mind-body techniques into one's routine may take time and dedication, but the benefits can be well worth it.

MEDITATION

Meditation is a practice that aims to achieve a state of relaxation and tranquillity by directing the focus of the mind towards a specific object, thought or activity. There are many different forms of meditation, but all involve focusing the mind and paying attention to the present moment. Meditation can lead to a state of relaxation and calmness. It is known to be effective in reducing levels of stress and anxiety, which can worsen chronic pain. It can also help you develop a more positive attitude towards your pain.

YOGA

Yoga is a physical and mental technique that combines different physical postures, breathing techniques, and mindfulness exercises. Yoga can improve flexibility, strength, and balance, as well as reduce stress and anxiety. Yoga can be adapted to accommodate your individual needs and abilities. It can also help you develop a sense of control over your body and pain.

TAI CHI

Tai chi is a technique of meditation with movement that involves slow, gentle movements and deep breathing. Tai chi can help improve balance, flexibility, strength, and reduce stress and anxiety. Like yoga, tai chi can be adapted to accommodate the needs and abilities of individuals with chronic pain.

OTHER MIND-BODY TECHNIQUES

There are many other mind-body techniques that can help manage chronic pain. These include progressive muscle relaxation, guided imagery, and biofeedback. These techniques can help to promote relaxation, decrease stress, and improve coping strategies.

INCORPORATING MIND-BODY TECHNIQUES

INTO YOUR PAIN MANAGEMENT PLAN

If you want to incorporate mind-body techniques into your pain management plan, you must approach the process with a willingness to try and be patient.

- Start with small steps. It can feel daunting and overwhelming if you are new to incorporating mind-body techniques into your pain management plan. Start with small, manageable steps, such as meditating for a few minutes daily or practising a few yoga poses. You can slowly increase the duration of your mind-body practices as you become more at ease with them.

- Experiment with different techniques. There are many different mind-body techniques to choose from, so it's essential to find the one that works best for you. Experiment with various methods until you find the ones that you enjoy and are effective in reducing your pain and improving your well-being.

- Be patient with yourself. Mind-body techniques require patience and practice. A period of time may pass before you notice the positive effects of these techniques. Take your time and be kind to yourself. Don't feel disheartened if you don't see any instant changes.

- Find a support system. Practising mind-body techniques can be challenging, especially if you're doing it on your own. Find a support system, such as a friend, family member, or support group, who can provide encouragement and motivation.

- Make it a habit. Consistency is essential when it comes to practising mind-body techniques. Make it a habit to incorporate these practices into your daily routine. Allocate a particular time every day for practising and ensure you adhere to it.

- Don't forget about the basics. Mind-body techniques are not a substitute for proper medical care. Ensure you also take care of the basics, like getting enough sleep, eating a healthy diet, and taking your medications as prescribed.

Remember, incorporating mind-body techniques into your pain management plan can be a powerful tool in reducing pain and improving overall well-being. With patience, practice, and the right support, you can find the techniques that work best for you and live beyond your pain.

CONCLUSION

Mind-body techniques can be a helpful addition to your pain management plan. These techniques can reduce pain intensity, improve physical functioning, and reduce depression and anxiety. Incorporating a variety of mind-body techniques into a pain management plan can be beneficial, as different techniques may work better for different individuals or at different times. It's essential to approach these techniques with patience and an open mind.

6. Managing Chronic Pain Through Meditation

A Beginner's Path to Inner Peace and Pain Relief

INTRODUCTION

Meditation is a practice that helps reduce pain, anxiety, and depression. This chapter will introduce meditation, including the benefits of meditation for chronic pain management, distinct types of meditation, and a step-by-step guide to getting started with meditation practice.

BENEFITS OF MEDITATION FOR CHRONIC PAIN MANAGEMENT

Meditation is a relaxation technique which can help improve chronic pain. Meditation has been found to be effective in reducing the intensity of pain, improving mood, and increasing the sense of well-being. In addition, meditation can help reduce pain perception by changing how the brain processes pain signals. By practising meditation, you can learn to relax your mind and body, which can help reduce stress and tension, leading to a reduction in pain.

ANALOGIES

Meditation can be compared to a fitness centre for the mind. Just as exercise strengthens and tones your muscles, meditation strengthens and tones your mind.

Meditation is like a mental shower. Just as a shower cleanses your body of dirt and sweat, meditation cleanses your mind of negative thoughts and emotions.

Meditation is like tending to a garden. Just as a gardener nurtures and cares for their plants, meditation helps you cultivate positive mental states and emotional resilience.

TYPES OF MEDITATION

There are several types of meditation practices that can be helpful for chronic pain management.

- Mindfulness meditation requires one to be fully present in the current moment and observe thoughts, emotions, and physical sensations without any judgment. The aim is to cultivate awareness and clarity of mind without getting entangled in the distractions of the past or future.

- Transcendental meditation is a mantra-based meditation technique where repeating a specific word or phrase is integral to the practice. This helps focus the mind and relax the body.

- Loving-kindness meditation is a form of meditation where individuals focus on cultivating feelings of love and kindness towards themselves and others. It can help reduce feelings of anger, resentment, and frustration, which can contribute to chronic pain.

GETTING STARTED WITH MEDITATION PRACTICE

Meditation practice can seem intimidating, but it's actually a simple practice that anyone can learn. One can initiate meditation by following these steps:

Select a quiet spot where you can meditate without any disturbances. Sit comfortably with your back straight and hands resting on your lap. Set a timer for 5-10 minutes. You can begin with a shorter period and slowly extend the length of your meditation sessions.

Pause briefly and shut your eyes while taking a deep breath; direct your attention towards the feeling of air going in and out of your body while you inhale and exhale.

Choose a meditation technique that feels comfortable for you. For example, you can try mindfulness meditation, loving-kindness meditation, or any other method that appeals to you.

Begin the meditation practice, focusing on your breath or the chosen technique. Whenever your mind starts to stray, softly redirect your focus back to your breathing or the meditation method selected.

When the timer rings, take a deep breath and gently open your eyes. Then, take a brief moment to think about your current emotional and physical state.

Consistency is vital when it comes to incorporating meditation into daily life. Regular practice is crucial for experiencing the full benefits of meditation.

USING MEDITATION IN YOUR PAIN MANAGEMENT PLAN

Here are a few suggestions for integrating meditation into your daily schedule:

- Start small: You don't need to meditate for prolonged periods to see benefits. Instead, start with just a few minutes a day and gradually increase the duration of your meditation sessions over time.

- Find a comfortable position: You can meditate in any position that feels comfortable, whether sitting in a chair, lying down, or even standing.

- Use props: Meditation cushions, blankets, or even chairs can help support the body and make the practice more comfortable.

- Incorporate movement: For those who find it challenging to sit still, incorporating movement into meditation can be helpful. For example, yoga, tai chi, or walking meditation can be effective.

- Focus on your breath: One way to focus your attention during meditation is by using your breath as an anchor. Whenever your mind starts to wander, bring your attention back to your breath.

- Don't judge yourself: You don't need to criticize yourself for your thoughts wandering during meditation since it's a common occurrence. When this happens, simply acknowledge it and gently bring your attention back to your breath. Don't judge yourself or get frustrated.

- Use guided meditations: If you're new to meditation, guided meditations can help you get started. There are many free apps and websites that help with guided meditations for beginners.

- Be consistent: Try to maintain consistency in your meditation practice by selecting a fixed time of day for it. Consistency is vital for setting up a meditation practice.

- Experiment with different times of the day: Try practising meditation at different times of the day to see what works best for you. Different individuals may have their preferred time of the day for meditation, with some finding it better to meditate in the morning while others prefer the evening.

- Be patient: Developing the skill of meditation requires patience and practice over time. So don't expect to see immediate results. However, with a consistent approach, you will gradually start to see improvements in your mental well-being.

- Seek support: Joining a meditation group or finding a teacher can support and guide your meditation practice.

- Incorporate mindfulness into daily activities, like eating, walking, and driving.

- Practice self-compassion: Chronic pain can be frustrating, and it's important to practice self-compassion. Recognize that meditation is a practice, and it's okay to have days where it's difficult to focus or stay present.

- Be open-minded: It's essential to have an open mind and try various meditation methods to discover which one is most effective for you, as there are numerous techniques available.

- Keep a journal: Keeping a journal of your meditation practice can help track progress and notice patterns or changes over time.

EASY STEPS FOR A MEDITATION TECHNIQUE

Here's a step-by-step guide for a simple meditation technique that can be helpful for chronic pain sufferers:

Body Scan Meditation:

It involves bringing attention to various parts of the body, noticing physical sensations, and cultivating awareness and relaxation. This technique can benefit people with chronic pain, as it allows them to focus their attention away from the pain and towards their body in a more positive way.

Step 1: Find a comfortable position, either sitting or lying down, where you can remain for the duration of the meditation. Make sure you are in a quiet, calming environment with minimal distractions.

Step 2: Start with deep breaths. Breathe in deeply through your nostrils and exhale through your mouth, repeating this a few times, and allow your body to relax with each exhale. You can also set a specific purpose for your practice, such as "I am letting go of tension and pain in my body" or "I am cultivating peace and relaxation."

Step 3: Bring attention to your toes. Focus your attention on your toes, noticing any physical sensations such as warmth, tingling, or tension. Don't judge or analyse these sensations; simply observe them with a curious and accepting attitude.

Step 4: Move up to your feet. Gradually move your attention up to your feet, noticing any sensations in your heels, arches, and tops of your feet. Keep breathing deeply and allow your feet to relax and release any tension.

Step 5: Move up to your legs. Continue moving your attention up to your legs, noticing any sensations in your calves, shins, and thighs. While you concentrate on each individual section of your body, imagine sending warmth and relaxation to that area.

Step 6: Focus on your hips and pelvis. Bring your attention to your hips and pelvis, noticing any sensations in your buttocks, lower back, and pelvic area. Allow any tension in this area to soften and release.

Step 7: Move up to your torso. Gradually move your attention up to your torso, noticing any sensations in your abdomen, chest, and back. Allow your breath to deepen and expand, and imagine sending love and kindness to your internal organs.

Step 8: Focus on your arms and hands. Shift your attention to your arms and hands, noticing any sensations in your fingers, palms, wrists, and forearms. Allow any tension in these areas to melt away with each exhale.

Step 9: Focus on your shoulders and neck. Bring your attention to your shoulders and neck, noticing any sensations in your shoulder blades, neck muscles, and jaw. Relax your shoulders and let them drop down from your ears. Also, try to loosen your jaw.

Step 10: End with a deep breath. Take a final deep breath, inhaling through your nose and exhaling through your mouth. Take a moment to feel the peace and relaxation in your body, and slowly open your eyes.

This meditation technique can be practised for a short duration of five minutes or extended up to 30 minutes, depending on your preference, schedule and needs. It's important to remember that meditation is a practice. Getting used to the process and seeing the benefits may take time.

CONCLUSION

Meditation is a simple and effective practice that can help manage chronic pain. By practising meditation regularly, individuals can learn to relax their minds and body, reducing stress and pain. However, it's important to remember that meditation takes time and patience. Still, regular practice can become a powerful tool in managing chronic pain.

7. Yoga for Chronic Pain

Empowerment Through the Power of Movement, Breath, and Mindfulness

INTRODUCTION

Practising yoga can be a powerful tool to help manage chronic pain. Yoga is a form of exercise that integrates physical poses, breathing exercises, and meditation. It focuses on the connection between the mind and the body to promote relaxation, reduce stress, and increase flexibility and strength. This chapter will explore the benefits of yoga for chronic pain and provide some tips and guidance for getting started.

THE BENEFITS OF YOGA FOR CHRONIC PAIN

Yoga has been shown to have several benefits for people with chronic pain, including:

- Reduced pain: Yoga can help reduce pain by increasing circulation, decreasing inflammation, and improving joint mobility.

- Improved mood: Yoga can elevate the secretion of endorphins, which function as natural analgesics, and alleviate stress and anxiety, thus enhancing mood.

- Increased strength and flexibility: Yoga practice has been found to enhance muscle strength and flexibility, which can help alleviate pain and reduce the risk of injury.

- Improved sleep: Yoga can help enhance sleep quality by

promoting relaxation and reducing stress.

GETTING STARTED WITH YOGA

If you are new to yoga, starting slowly and listening to your body is essential. Here are some suggestions to begin the process:

Choose a class: Look for a yoga class specifically designed for people with chronic pain or beginners. Speak with the instructor beforehand to discuss any concerns you may have and ask about modifications for specific poses. They can help create a customised yoga practice that is safe and effective for you.

Wear comfortable clothing which will allow you to move freely and comfortably.

Use props: Yoga props, such as blocks and straps, can be helpful for modifying poses and making them more accessible.

Focus on the breath: Pay attention to your breath during your yoga practice. Deep, slow breathing can help promote relaxation and reduce pain.

Practice self-compassion and patience. It's important to remember that yoga is a journey, and it may take time to see the benefits. Try not to exert yourself excessively and pay attention to any signals of pain or discomfort your body may be sending.

Incorporate mindfulness and meditation practices into your yoga routine. These practices can aid in the reduction of stress and anxiety, which can worsen pain.

Experiment with different types of yoga to find what works best for you. Gentle yoga, restorative yoga, and yin yoga may be particularly beneficial for people with chronic pain.

Don't compare yourself to others in your yoga class or on social media. Each individual is unique, and a treatment or method that is effective for one person may not necessarily be effective for another. Instead, focus on your own progress and listen to your body's needs.

Take breaks and rest when needed. It's okay to change or skip certain poses if they are causing pain or discomfort. Remember that yoga is meant to be a practice of self-care, not self-punishment.

Regular practice is crucial to experience the advantages of yoga. You can begin by dedicating a small part of your day to the training and gradually extend the duration as you become more comfortable.

EASY STEPS FOR YOGA

You can use the following stepwise approach to performing yoga poses that can help alleviate chronic pain in different regions of the body:

Neck Pain:

a. Start with the Cat-Cow pose:

Assume a position with your hands and knees touching the ground. Make sure to position your hands and knees in a way that your wrists are directly beneath your shoulders and your knees are aligned under your hips. Take a deep breath in, allowing your back to gently curve and lifting your head and tailbone upwards (Cow pose). As you exhale, round your spine by gently curving it inward and tuck your chin towards your chest (Cat pose). Repeat this sequence for a few breaths.

b. Move into the Thread the Needle pose:

From the Cat pose, slide your right arm under your left arm and lower your right shoulder and ear to the mat. Maintain this pose for a few breaths, allowing your body to relax and adjust. Afterwards, you can switch sides or move on to the next pose as needed.

Shoulder Pain:

a. Begin with the Eagle Arms pose:

Extend your arms forward, reaching them out in front of you. Gently cross your left arm over your right, and bring your palms together, creating a prayer-like position in front of your chest. This would create a gentle stretch in your shoulders and upper back. Bend your elbows and lift your forearms, bringing your fingertips toward the ceiling. Maintain this crossed-arm position with palms together and hold it for a few breaths, allowing the stretch to deepen. Afterwards, release the arms, switch sides, and repeat the same sequence with the right arm crossing over the left.

b. Practice the Cow Face pose:

Extend your right arm to the side, bend your elbow, and reach your right hand behind your back. Then, stretch your left arm overhead, bend your elbow, and extend your left hand behind your back. If possible, clasp your fingers together. Maintain this position for a few breaths, then switch sides.

Elbow Pain:

a. Start with the Downward Facing Dog pose:

Assume a position with your hands and knees touching the ground, then lift your knees off the ground and gently straighten your legs, forming an inverted V shape with your body. Keep your elbows slightly bent. Hold for a few breaths.

b. Move into the Forearm Plank pose:

Lower down onto your forearms, aligning your elbows directly under your shoulders. Try to maintain your body in a straight line from head to heels, engaging your core muscles. Hold for a few breaths.

Back pain:

a. Begin with the Child's pose:

Kneel on the floor, touch your big toes together, and sit on your heels. Extend your arms forward, reaching them out in front of you, and gently lower your forehead towards the mat. Allow your upper body to relax and rest in this position, feeling a gentle stretch in your shoulders and a sense of grounding. Maintain and relax in this position for a few breaths.

b. Practice the Bridge pose:

Lie down on your back and bend your knees, bringing them towards your chest. Place your feet flat on the floor, ensuring they are hip-width apart and parallel to each other. This position allows for a relaxed and stable base as you move into other poses or focus to release tension in your lower back. Engage your feet and press them firmly into the mat. At the same time, press your arms down into the mat, creating a sense of grounding and activating the muscles in your legs and arms. This action helps to stabilize your body, and now try to lift your hips and interlace your fingers beneath your pelvis. Hold for a few breaths.

Abdominal pain:

a. Start with the Cobra pose:

Lie on your stomach, place your palms on the mat beside your shoulders, and press the tops of your feet into the mat. Inhale and gently lift your chest off the ground, keeping your lower ribs on the floor. Hold for a few breaths.

b. Move into the Supine Twist pose:

Lie down on your back and draw your knees towards your chest. Extend your arms out to the sides, forming a "T" shape. While keeping your shoulders grounded, lower your knees to the right side of your body. Hold this position for a few breaths, allowing a gentle stretch to occur. Then, switch sides by bringing your knees back to the centre and lowering them to the left side. Remember to maintain steady and relaxed breathing throughout the movement.

Hip Pain:

a. Begin with the Pigeon pose:

Assume a high plank position, and then bring your right knee forward and position it behind your right wrist. Gently extend your left leg straight behind you while keeping your hips square. Lower your upper body onto your forearms or onto the mat. Maintain this pose for a few breaths, allowing for a gentle stretch. Afterwards, switch sides by releasing the pose and repeating the sequence with the opposite leg.

b. Practice the Butterfly pose:

Take a seat on the floor and gently bend your knees, bringing the soles of your feet together. Allow your knees to gently open out to the sides as much as comfortably possible, creating a diamond shape with your legs. This provides a gentle stretch for the inner thighs and groin area. Hold onto your feet or ankles, lengthen your spine, and gently press your knees toward the ground. Hold for a few breaths.

Knee Pain:

a. Start with the Standing Forward Bend pose:

Stand with your feet positioned hip-width apart. From there, hinge forward at the hips, allowing your upper body to fold forward and hang down towards the floor. In order to relive pressure on the knees, you can keep your knees slightly bent. In this pose, you release tension in the hamstrings and the back of the body while promoting a sense of relaxation. Hold for a few breaths.

b. Move into the Reclining Hand-to-Big-Toe pose:

Lie down on your back and gently raise your right leg up towards the ceiling. Grasp your right big toe using your right hand, maintaining a comfortable grip. Your left leg can remain extended on the floor or, if desired, you can bend it with the foot resting flat on the ground. Maintain this posture for a few breaths, allowing the gentle stretch in the back of your leg to be felt. Then, release the pose and switch sides by repeating the sequence with your left leg.

Ankle Pain:

a. Begin with the Downward Facing Dog pose:

Follow the instructions provided in the shoulder pain section.

b. Practice the Reclining Hand-to-Big-Toe pose:

Follow the instructions provided in the knee pain section.

It is crucial to be mindful and take notice of your body's signals and modify the poses as needed. Never push yourself into pain or discomfort. Depending on your preference and comfort level, these poses can be practised in sequence or individually. Remember to breathe deeply and focus on relaxing your body as you move through the poses. Gradually build your practice and be patient with your progress.

HOW TO MODIFY YOGA POSES WHEN IN PAIN

You can use the following practical tips and modifications to make yoga poses more accessible with chronic pain:

- Use props: Props such as yoga blocks, bolsters, blankets, and straps can provide support and make poses more comfortable. For example, using a block under your hands in the Forward Bend pose can help individuals with tight hamstrings or lower back pain.

- Modify the range of motion: Reduce the range of motion in poses to avoid exacerbating pain. As an illustration, when practising the Pigeon pose, you have the option to place a block or a folded blanket under the hip of the bent leg. This modification helps to reduce the intensity of the stretch, allowing for a more comfortable and accessible experience.

- Focus on alignment: Pay attention to proper alignment in each pose. This helps distribute the workload and reduce strain on specific areas. A certified yoga instructor can guide you in aligning your body correctly.

- Practice gentle variations: Opt for gentler variations of poses that are less intense. For instance, instead of the full Cobra pose, you can try a Baby Cobra by keeping your forearms on the ground and gently lifting your chest.

- Modify weight-bearing poses: If weight-bearing poses are challenging, you can perform them with the support of a chair or against a wall. For example, a Wall Dog pose can be done by standing a few feet away from a wall, firmly placing your hands on the wall, and walking your feet back to form a diagonal line.

- Use modifications for seated poses: If sitting on the floor is uncomfortable, sit on a cushion or a folded blanket to elevate your hips. This can alleviate strain on the lower back and hips. Chairs can also be used for support in seated poses.

- Practice mindful breathing: Incorporate deep, mindful breathing into your practice. Focusing on your breath can help relax the body and mind, reducing pain and tension.

- Seek guidance from a professional: Consider working with a certified yoga instructor or a qualified physical therapist with experience in helping individuals dealing with chronic pain. They can provide personalised modifications and adaptations based on your specific needs.

CONCLUSION

Yoga has the potential to serve as an effective method for coping with persistent pain and enhancing one's overall well-being. By reducing pain, improving mood, increasing strength and flexibility, and improving sleep, yoga can help you feel better both physically and mentally. By following these tips and practising regularly, you can begin to experience the benefits of yoga for chronic pain.

8. Tai Chi for Managing Chronic Pain

A Beginner's Guide

INTRODUCTION

Tai Chi is a type of low-impact physical activity that originated in China and has been practised for centuries. It involves slow, flowing movements designed to promote balance, flexibility, and relaxation. It is a type of exercise that has a low impact on the body and can be customised to accommodate individuals of varying fitness levels and ages, making it a safe and accessible choice for many individuals.

HOW DOES TAI CHI HELP PAIN?

Tai Chi is believed to help reduce chronic pain by promoting relaxation and reducing stress, which can often worsen pain symptoms. In addition, it has been shown to improve balance, coordination, and flexibility, thereby decreasing the possibility of falls and subsequent injuries that could worsen pain and improve your overall physical and mental well-being.

Tai Chi can effectively decrease pain and improve the quality of life in people with various chronic pain conditions. If you are new to Tai Chi, starting slowly and working at your own pace is essential.

EASY STEPS FOR TAI CHI

Below are some uncomplicated actions to start your journey:

- Step 1: Find a comfortable place to practice. It is vital to find a quiet, comfortable place where you can practice Tai

Chi without any distractions. Ideally, this would be a quiet room or a peaceful outdoor space where you can focus on your movements and your breath.

◦ Step 2: Wear comfortable clothing. When practising Tai Chi, it is important to wear loose, comfortable clothing that enables ease of movement. This will help you to move more freely without any restrictions or discomfort.

◦ Step 3: Begin with warm-up exercises. Before beginning your Tai Chi routine, it is essential to do some gentle warm-up exercises to help prepare your body for movement. Some good warm-up exercises include shoulder shrugs, neck stretches, and leg swings.

◦ Step 4: Learn the basic Tai Chi movements. Tai Chi movements are slow and gentle, designed to promote relaxation and balance.

◦ Step 5: Practice regularly. Practising regularly is essential to get the most benefit from Tai Chi. Aim to practice for at least 10-15 minutes a day, and gradually extend the duration of your sessions as you become more at ease with the movements.

BASIC TAI CHI MOVEMENTS

You can try the following basic Tai Chi movements that may help with pain in different joints.

Wu Ji:

Stand with your feet shoulder-width apart, parallel to each other. Distribute your weight evenly on both feet. This stance promotes a grounded and centred posture, which can help alleviate pain in the knees, ankles, and hips.

Horse Stance (Ma Bu):

Start with your feet wider than shoulder-width apart and slightly turned out. Gently bend your knees and sink your hips down as if sitting on an imaginary chair. This stance strengthens the legs and can provide relief for knee and hip pain.

Bow Stance (Gong Bu):

Take a step forward with one foot, keeping the distance between your feet wider than shoulder-width apart. Gently bend your front knee while keeping your back leg straight. This stance helps strengthen the legs and can assist with knee, hip, and ankle pain.

Empty Stance (Xu Bu):

Take a step forward with one foot, keeping the majority of your body weight on your back leg. Keep the front foot lightly touching the ground. This stance helps improve balance and can benefit ankle and knee pain.

Cloud Hands (Yun Shou):

Stand with your feet shoulder-width apart. Visualise yourself holding a big ball in front of your torso. Shift your weight from side to side, allowing your arms to follow the movement. This gentle twisting motion can help relieve shoulder, elbow, and wrist pain.

Single Whip (Dan Bian):

Start in a neutral standing position, then step forward with one foot, keeping your feet wider than shoulder-width apart. Rotate your body, extend one arm forward, and turn the other hand outward. This stance can help promote flexibility in the wrists and relieve shoulder and elbow pain.

PRACTICAL TIPS AND MODIFICATIONS WHEN IN PAIN

Here are some practical tips and modifications for individuals with pain in specific joints when practising the above Tai Chi stances:

Wu Ji:

Modify the stance width: Adjust the width of your feet to find a position that feels comfortable for your joints. You can start with a narrower stance and gradually widen it as you build strength and flexibility.

Use support: If needed, you can practice Wu Ji with the support of a chair or against a wall to help maintain balance and reduce strain on the joints.

Horse Stance:

Partial squat: If bending your knees deeply causes discomfort, you can modify the stance by performing a partial squat. Bend your knees to a degree that feels comfortable for your joints, gradually increasing the depth as your flexibility improves.

Use support: If balance is an issue, practice Horse Stance with the support of a chair or wall to provide stability and reduce stress on the knees and hips.

Bow Stance:

Reduce the stance length: Shorten the distance between your feet to decrease the depth of the lunge. Find a position where you feel a gentle stretch without causing pain or discomfort.

Use support: If needed, place your hands on a wall or chair for balance and support during the Bow Stance, especially if you have instability or pain in the knees and hips.

Empty Stance:

Step with caution: When stepping forward into the Empty Stance, take small and controlled steps to minimise strain on the joints. You can slowly expand the range of motion as you become more comfortable and flexible.

Decrease weight shift: Instead of fully shifting your body weight onto the front foot, keep a larger portion of your weight on the back leg to reduce pressure on the front knee and ankle.

Cloud Hands:

Reduce arm movement: If you experience discomfort in the

shoulders or elbows, decrease the range of motion in the arms during the Cloud Hands movement. Focus on gentle and controlled movements without overstretching.

Modify hand position: If needed, soften the hand position by keeping the fingers relaxed instead of fully extending them, which can help alleviate strain in the wrists and fingers.

Single Whip:

Adapt arm extension: If extending the arm fully causes discomfort in the shoulders or elbows, modify the extension by bending the arm slightly. Find a position that allows for a comfortable stretch without aggravating the pain.

Slow and controlled movement: Perform the Single Whip movement at a slower pace, emphasising control and proper alignment to help reduce the strain on the joints and promote stability.

It's essential to work within your comfort zone and not push into pain. Consulting with a qualified Tai Chi instructor or physical therapist can provide further personalised guidance and modifications based on your specific condition.

CONCLUSION

Tai Chi has been shown to offer many benefits for helping with chronic pain. From improving physical functioning and reducing pain intensity to lowering stress and anxiety, Tai Chi is a mild and efficient type of physical activity that can be performed by individuals of any age and ability. In addition, Tai Chi is a suitable exercise for individuals with chronic pain, as it is a low-impact activity which is gentle on the joints and muscles. This is especially beneficial for people who may find it challenging to engage in more intense exercises due to their pain. Finally, by incorporating Tai Chi into a comprehensive pain management plan, you can experience improved physical and mental health, improving your quality of life.

9. Nutrition and Chronic Pain

Understanding the Role of Diet in Pain Management and Inflammation Reduction

INTRODUCTION

Chronic pain can be a complex condition, and numerous elements can contribute to its occurrence and continuity. One of these factors is nutrition. Diet plays a crucial role in managing pain and reducing inflammation in the body. This chapter will explore the link between nutrition and chronic pain and discuss how making dietary changes can help to manage pain and improve overall health.

UNDERSTANDING INFLAMMATION

When the body experiences an injury, infection or any other form of damage, inflammation is a common natural response. Long-term inflammation can play a role in the creation and endurance of prolonged pain. Specific types of food can instigate inflammation within the body, but certain foods may assist in decreasing inflammation. To comprehend the impact of inflammation on long-term pain, it's crucial to understand its role in the body, as this can help guide dietary choices.

THE ROLE OF NUTRIENTS IN PAIN MANAGEMENT

Proper nutrition, including vitamins, minerals, and omega-3 fatty acids, is essential in managing chronic pain. For example, vitamin D is vital for bone health and may help to reduce chronic pain. Omega-3 fatty acids, found in foods like flaxseed and fish, have been shown to reduce inflammation and improve pain symptoms in some people with chronic pain. One potential benefit of vitamin B12 is its ability to alleviate nerve pain, while magnesium may help to relieve muscle pain and cramps. A well-rounded diet that provides a range of nutrients is crucial for promoting general health and managing pain.

ANALOGY

Think of your body as a car. Similar to how a car requires fuel to operate efficiently, your body needs food to perform at its optimal level. Choosing the right fuel (i.e., healthy, nutrient-dense foods) can help your body function better and reduce pain and inflammation.

BENEFITS OF A WHOLE FOODS DIET

A whole foods diet emphasises minimally processed, nutrient-dense foods. This type of diet can help to reduce inflammation and support overall health. A whole foods diet should consist of a variety of foods, including whole grains and lean proteins, to support overall health and pain management. You can lessen inflammation and enhance pain symptoms by steering clear of processed foods and those with high amounts of sugar and unhealthy fats.

IMPORTANCE OF BALANCED MACRONUTRIENT INTAKE

While it's essential to consume various nutrients, it's also important to balance the intake of macronutrients - protein, carbohydrates, and fat. Each macronutrient has a distinct role in the body, and an imbalance in intake can contribute to inflammation and pain. For example, excessive intake of refined carbohydrates and sugar can lead to insulin resistance and inflammation, while insufficient protein intake can contribute to muscle weakness and pain.

IMPORTANCE OF HYDRATION

Staying hydrated would help your overall health and pain management. Water is essential for proper body function and can help to reduce inflammation. Try to consume a minimum of 8-10 cups of water daily. Avoid sugary drinks and excessive caffeine, which can contribute to dehydration. Some practical tips to stay hydrated throughout the day include carrying a water bottle, scheduling alerts or notifications to remind yourself to drink water at specific intervals throughout the day and including hydrating foods such as watermelon and cucumber in your diet.

FOODS TO INCLUDE IN YOUR DIET

Many foods could be beneficial for people with chronic pain. For example, ginger and turmeric are spices that have anti-inflammatory properties and can help decrease pain. In addition, consuming foods that contain high levels of omega-3 fatty acids, such as walnuts and tuna, may also offer benefits for pain management. Furthermore, vegetables with dark green leaves, like spinach and kale, are abundant in essential nutrients that contribute to general well-being.

FOODS TO AVOID

When managing chronic pain, it can be beneficial to be mindful of certain foods that may exacerbate inflammation or trigger pain responses in the body. While individual sensitivities may vary, it is generally recommended to limit or avoid processed foods high in refined sugars, trans fats, and artificial additives. Additionally, some people find that reducing their intake of inflammatory foods such as red meat, processed meats, refined grains, and high-fat dairy products can help alleviate symptoms. Reducing the intake of caffeine, alcohol, and foods with excessive additives and preservatives could also be advantageous. Maintaining a food diary and paying attention to how certain foods affect your pain levels can help identify specific triggers and guide you in making informed dietary choices that support your overall well-being and pain management efforts.

PRACTICAL TIPS FOR MAKING DIETARY CHANGES

Making dietary changes can be challenging, but it is essential for managing chronic pain and improving overall health. Some practical tips include planning meals in advance, shopping for whole foods, and preparing meals at home.

Avoid skipping meals: Skipping meals can lead to blood sugar drops, worsening pain and inflammation. Instead, try to eat regular, well-rounded meals throughout the day.

Mindful eating: Eating mindfully can help you to better tune in to your body's hunger and fullness cues and to make more intentional food choices. This can be particularly helpful for those who struggle with emotional eating or have difficulty identifying the specific foods that trigger their pain.

Collaborate with a healthcare professional or a licensed nutritionist: If you're unsure which foods to eat or avoid or how to create a healthy eating plan, consider working with a healthcare professional or a licensed nutritionist who can provide guidance and support.

POTENTIAL BENEFITS OF A PLANT-BASED DIET

A plant-based diet, which is high in fruits, whole grains, vegetables, and legumes, may be beneficial for reducing pain and inflammation in some people with chronic pain. This type of diet is rich in antioxidants and anti-inflammatory compounds. In addition, it may help to balance the body's microbiome, which plays a crucial role in immune function and inflammation.

IMPACT OF FOOD PREPARATION METHODS

The way in which food is prepared can also impact its nutrient content and potential to trigger inflammation. For example, frying and grilling can produce harmful compounds that contribute to inflammation, while steaming and baking are gentler cooking methods that may help to preserve the nutrient content of foods.

NUTRIENTS THAT MAY HELP ALLEVIATE CHRONIC PAIN

Vitamin B12:

Vitamin B12 is a necessary nutrient that has a significant function in the proper functioning of nerves and may help reduce nerve pain. However, it can be challenging for vegetarians and vegans to get enough of this nutrient as it is primarily found in animal products. Some food sources of vitamin B12 include meat such as beef, liver, and chicken; fish like salmon, trout, and tuna; dairy products such as milk, cheese, yoghurt, and eggs; and fortified breakfast cereals and plant-based milk alternatives like soy and almond milk.

Magnesium:

It is a crucial mineral that has a significant impact on muscle and nerve function, and it has been found to help alleviate muscle pain and cramps. To obtain an ample amount of magnesium, it's recommended to consume foods such as green leafy vegetables like spinach, kale, and Swiss chard, nuts and seeds like almonds, cashews, and pumpkin seeds, whole grains like barley, brown rice and quinoa, legumes like lentils and chickpeas, and even avocado. These foods are a great source of magnesium and adding them to your diet can help minimise muscle pain and cramps.

Vitamin D:

It is not only essential for maintaining bone health, but it also contributes to managing chronic pain. Individuals with chronic pain may experience higher levels of pain and reduced quality of life when they have insufficient levels of vitamin D. Vitamin D is crucial for managing the immune system and alleviating inflammation, which may be a contributing factor to pain. Foods that are rich sources of vitamin D include oily fish like salmon, tuna, sardines and mackerel, as well as dairy products fortified with vitamin D, such as yoghurt and cereals fortified with this nutrient. It can also be obtained from exposure to sunlight, but this can be difficult to achieve in some climates or during certain times of the year.

Omega-3 Fatty Acids:

They belong to the category of unsaturated fats that have been demonstrated to have numerous health advantages, such as reducing inflammation and enhancing heart health. In addition, increasing omega-3 intake can reduce pain and stiffness in people with chronic pain conditions such as rheumatoid arthritis and osteoarthritis. Omega-3s are found in oily fish like sardines, mackerel, salmon, cod liver oil and tuna, as well as in nuts and plant-based sources such as flaxseed, chia seeds, and walnuts.

WHOLE FOOD MEAL PLANS

Here are a few examples of nutritious and pain-friendly whole foods meal plans and recipes:

Mediterranean Diet Meal Plan:

Opting for a Mediterranean-style diet is a beneficial choice for those looking for a pain-friendly meal plan that is also nutritious. Here's a sample meal plan for the day:

For breakfast, try having a serving of Greek yoghurt topped with various mixed berries and a small number of nuts for added texture and nutrition.

Snack: Carrots and hummus.

Lunch: A mixture of greens, cucumber, tomato, and avocado with grilled chicken to prepare a salad.

A healthy snack option could be sliced apples served with almond butter.

For dinner, you could have some baked salmon paired with roasted vegetables (such as bell peppers, zucchini, and eggplant).

Anti-Inflammatory Smoothie:

This smoothie is a quick and easy way to get some anti-inflammatory nutrients into your diet:

1 cup frozen mixed berries

1 banana

1/2 cup plain Greek yoghurt

1/2 cup unsweetened almond milk

1 tablespoon chia seeds

1 teaspoon honey

Blend all ingredients together until smooth.

Quinoa Salad:

This hearty salad is packed with anti-inflammatory ingredients:

1 cup cooked quinoa

1/2 cup black beans

1/2 cup chopped cherry tomatoes

1/2 avocado, diced

1/4 cup chopped fresh cilantro

Juice of 1 lime

Salt and pepper to taste

Mix the above ingredients in a bowl and serve.

Roasted Vegetable and Chicken Sheet Pan Dinner:

This sheet pan dinner is an excellent option for an easy, one-pan meal:

1 pound boneless, skinless chicken thighs

2 cups chopped vegetables (such as sweet potato, broccoli, and red onion)

1 tablespoon olive oil

1 teaspoon dried thyme

Salt and pepper to taste

Preheat oven to 400°F. Toss the chicken and vegetables with olive oil, thyme, salt, and pepper. Spread on a sheet pan and roast for 25-30 minutes until the chicken is fully cooked and the vegetables are tender.

These are just a few examples of pain-friendly meals and recipes. By focusing on whole, nutrient-dense foods and incorporating anti-inflammatory ingredients, you can create a healthy and delicious diet that supports your overall health and wellness.

While supplements and specific "superfoods" may have some anti-inflammatory properties, it is essential not to rely solely on them for pain management. These supplements and foods may be beneficial but should not be viewed as a magic bullet for pain relief. It is crucial to remember that a balanced and varied whole-food diet is the foundation for any dietary changes aimed at reducing pain and inflammation. Additionally, taking high doses of supplements can be harmful and even toxic in some cases.

Furthermore, focusing too much on individual nutrients may distract from the importance of a well-rounded diet. A well-balanced diet must consist of an assortment of wholesome foods, including fruits, vegetables, whole grains, lean protein sources, and nourishing fats. These foods contain a complex mix of nutrients and phytochemicals that work together to support your overall health and reduce inflammation.

CONCLUSION

Nutrition plays a crucial role in managing chronic pain and reducing inflammation. A whole foods diet that emphasises nutrient-dense, minimally processed foods can help to reduce pain symptoms and improve overall health. It is essential to avoid foods that trigger inflammation and to stay hydrated. With some practical tips and support, making dietary changes can be a manageable and effective way to manage chronic pain.

While supplements and specific foods may have some benefits in reducing pain and inflammation, they should be viewed as a complement to a balanced and varied whole foods diet. It is important to prioritise a healthy and balanced diet as the foundation for pain management.

10. Transcutaneous Electrical Nerve Stimulation

Exploring TENS Machines for Chronic Pain Relief

INTRODUCTION

For individuals struggling with chronic pain, finding effective pain management techniques is essential for maintaining their quality of life. Transcutaneous Electrical Nerve Stimulation (TENS) has become increasingly popular among the many treatment options. TENS machines are portable, small devices that use low-voltage electrical currents to help alleviate pain. In this chapter, we will explore how TENS machines work, how they can benefit those dealing with chronic pain, as well as potential risks to be aware of when using TENS for pain management.

WHAT IS A TENS MACHINE?

It is a small portable, battery-operated device that uses electrodes to deliver electrical impulses to the skin's surface. These electrical impulses stimulate the nerves and interfere with pain signals travelling to the brain. TENS machines are usually powered by batteries and offer adjustable features that enable users to personalise the intensity, duration, and frequency of the electrical signals.

HOW DOES IT HELP CHRONIC PAIN?

The TENS machine functions by activating the sensory nerves, thereby impeding the transmission of pain signals to the brain. The electrical impulses also encourage the production of endorphins, which are the body's natural painkillers. TENS machines can be utilised on their own or in conjunction with other methods for managing pain. TENS machines are non-invasive and can be used at home or on the go, making them a convenient choice for individuals with chronic pain.

BENEFITS OF TENS MACHINES FOR CHRONIC PAIN

TENS machines offer several benefits for chronic pain management. They are non-invasive and drug-free, making them an attractive option for people who prefer to avoid medication. TENS machines are also relatively inexpensive and easy to use, making them accessible to a wide range of people.

TENS machines are effective in managing various types of chronic pain, including back pain, arthritis and fibromyalgia. The electrical impulses delivered by the TENS machine can help reduce pain, improve circulation, and relax muscles. Some people also report that TENS machines help them sleep better and improve their overall mood.

RISKS OF TENS MACHINES FOR CHRONIC PAIN

While TENS machines are generally considered safe, there are some risks associated with their use. Individuals with specific health conditions like epilepsy should refrain from using TENS machines. The electrical impulses delivered by the TENS machine can also cause skin irritation rarely. It's crucial to carefully follow the instructions for the TENS machine and use it as directed. Patients with pacemakers or other implanted devices should consult with their doctor before using a TENS machine, as the electrical impulses can interfere with these devices. TENS machines are not recommended while you are driving a car.

It is important to note that TENS machines do not work for everyone and may not provide complete pain relief. In addition, the effectiveness of TENS can vary depending on the individual's condition and pain level. Additionally, it is essential to note that

TENS machines should not be used as a replacement for medical care and should be used as a complementary therapy to other pain management techniques.

USING A TENS MACHINE FOR CHRONIC PAIN

When using a TENS machine for chronic pain, the placement of the electrodes is crucial for maximum effectiveness. The location of the pain will determine where the electrodes should be placed. Here are some general guidelines for placing the electrodes in different areas of chronic pain:

- Neck pain: Place one to two pairs of electrodes on either side of your spine in the back of your neck at the level of pain.
- Shoulder pain: Place the electrodes in the front and back of your shoulder. Alternatively, the pads can also be placed at the top of the shoulder and in the muscle bulk above your shoulder blade.

- Wrist pain: Place one electrode on the front of the wrist and the other on the back of the wrist.

- Back pain: Place two electrodes on either side of the spine at the level of the pain.

- Abdominal pain: Place one electrode on either side of the spine at the level of the pain and the other electrode on the abdomen at the level of the pain.

- Hip pain: Place one electrode on the front of the hip and the other on the back of the hip.

- Knee pain: Position one pair of electrodes above the knee, on either side and another pair of electrodes below the knee, on either side.

It is essential to understand that these instructions are not specific to every individual and may vary depending on personal circumstances. It is advised to initially begin with a low-intensity level and gradually increase the intensity until a strong but comfortable sensation is felt.

EASY STEPS TO USE TENS

The following is a set of instructions outlining the steps to properly use a TENS machine:

- First, ensure that the TENS machine is switched off and that you have read the manufacturer's instructions.

- Locate the electrodes that come with the TENS machine. These are usually sticky pads with a small metal stud in the middle.

- Identify the area where you will be placing the electrodes. This will depend on where you are experiencing pain.

- Before placing the electrodes, cleaning the area thoroughly to eliminate any oils or lotions is essential. This helps ensure good contact and better results.

- Dry the area thoroughly before proceeding.

- Peel off the protective backing on the electrodes to reveal the sticky side.

- Place the electrodes on the skin, making sure they are correctly positioned. Normally we use two electrodes at a time and sometimes four electrodes. The electrodes should be placed on either side of the area where you are experiencing pain. For example, if you have lower back pain, electrodes should be placed on either side of your spine.

- Spacing between electrodes: Keep the electrodes a few inches apart from each other. This allows the electrical stimulation to cover a wider area and potentially provide better pain relief.

- Once the electrodes are in place, connect them to the

TENS machine. The machine will have two lead wires that connect to the electrodes. Ensure that the wires are firmly attached.

- Turn on the TENS machine and select the settings that are appropriate for your needs. There will be different settings for intensity, frequency, and pulse width. Begin with a low level of intensity and slowly raise it until you experience a strong yet tolerable feeling. This helps you find the right level of stimulation that effectively reduces your pain without causing discomfort.

- Adjusting for comfort: You can adjust the placement of the electrodes slightly to find the most comfortable position for you. Experiment with small movements to ensure they are in a spot that feels good.

- Trial and error: It's important to remember that electrode placement can vary depending on the individual and their specific pain condition. It might take some trial and error to find the optimal placement that works best for you.

- Keep the TENS machine on for the recommended duration, usually around 30 - 60 minutes. After the session, turn off the machine and remove the electrodes.

- If you experience any adverse effects or the pain worsens, discontinue use and consult with a healthcare professional.

- Clean the electrodes with a damp cloth and store them in a cool, dry place.

- Make sure to follow the instructions that come with the machine and consult with a healthcare professional if you have any concerns.

CONCLUSION

TENS machines can be a valuable tool for managing chronic pain, but they are not suitable for everyone. However, with proper use, TENS machines can provide relief from chronic pain and improve your quality of life.

11. Cognitive Behavioural Therapy (CBT)

Strategies for Cognitive Restructuring and Behaviour Modification

INTRODUCTION

Chronic pain can affect various areas of an individual's life. For example, it may have a substantial impact on daily activities, work, social relationships, and overall well-being, from your physical health to your emotional well-being. One practical approach for managing chronic pain is cognitive-behavioural therapy (CBT). It is a talk therapy that helps individuals change their thoughts and behaviours to better manage their pain. This chapter will discuss CBT, how it works, and some strategies you can use to help manage your chronic pain.

WHAT IS CBT?

Cognitive behavioural therapy (CBT) is a form of psychotherapy which is based on the idea that our thoughts, feelings, and behaviours are interconnected. Specifically, CBT posits that our thoughts and beliefs about our circumstances can influence our emotional reactions and behavioural responses. For example, CBT for pain management involves identifying negative thought patterns and ideas about pain and challenging and reframing those thoughts more positively and realistically. Through this process, individuals with chronic pain can develop new coping strategies to better manage pain-related behaviours and improve their psychological well-being and quality of life. CBT has effectively treated a range of mental health and medical conditions, including chronic pain, anxiety, and depression.

HOW DOES CBT WORK?

In the context of managing chronic pain, CBT entails recognising and disputing negative thoughts and attitudes concerning pain. These negative thoughts can lead to feelings of hopelessness and despair and may contribute to a cycle of pain and disability. Negative thoughts and behaviours can also contribute to the intensity and persistence of pain.

In CBT, these negative thoughts are reframed more positively. CBT may also help you to develop coping strategies for managing pain-related behaviours, such as pacing and goal setting.

COGNITIVE RESTRUCTURING FOR CHRONIC PAIN MANAGEMENT

One of the main strategies used in CBT for pain management is cognitive restructuring. For example, an individual may think, "I can't do anything because of my pain." With the help of CBT, the individual can learn to challenge this thought by reframing it to, "While I may not be able to do everything I used to, there are still things I can do to improve my quality of life." Individuals can reduce emotional distress and pain intensity by changing negative thought patterns.

Here's a breakdown of what it involves.

Identify negative thoughts:

The first step is to identify negative thoughts or beliefs that you have about your pain. Negative thoughts are ideas about your pain that are not helpful and can make you feel more anxious, sad, or frustrated and even worsen your pain. The first step in changing these negative thoughts is identifying them and becoming aware of how they affect you.

I have given some examples of negative thoughts related to

chronic pain that can be addressed with cognitive-behavioural therapy (CBT) below.

Catastrophising: "This pain is unbearable and will never go away. I'm never going to be able to live a regular life."

Overgeneralisation: "I've had this pain for so long, it's never going to get better. Nothing I do will make a difference."

All-or-nothing thinking: "If I can't do everything I used to do before the pain started, then there's no point in doing anything at all."

Personalisation: "My pain is all my fault. If I had taken better care of myself, I wouldn't be in this situation."

Mind-reading: "Other people think I'm weak or lazy because I can't do certain things because of my pain."

Catastrophic thinking: "If I push myself too hard, I'll make the pain worse and never be able to recover."

Evaluate the evidence:

Once you've identified these negative thoughts, evaluating the evidence for and against them is essential. For example, if you believe that you can't do anything because of your pain, consider times when you have been able to do things despite the pain.

Challenge negative thoughts:

The next step involves disputing pessimistic thoughts and convictions and substituting them with more pragmatic and optimistic ones. This can include asking yourself, "Is this thought based on facts or assumptions?" and "Is there evidence to support this thought?"

Practice new thoughts:

Once you've identified and challenged negative thoughts, it's important to practice new thoughts and beliefs regularly. This can involve repeating positive affirmations, visualising positive outcomes, and reminding yourself of past successes.

In the next few paragraphs, I have given some examples of pragmatic and positive thoughts that can help manage chronic pain as part of CBT.

Catastrophising: "This pain is challenging, but I am taking steps to manage it, and it will eventually improve. I will work towards living a fulfilling life despite my pain."

Overgeneralisation: "Although I have had pain for a while, I can try different treatments to see what works best for me. There is hope for improvement, and I can take control of my pain."

All-or-nothing thinking: "I can still do many things that I enjoy, even if I can't do everything I used to do. I will focus on what I can rather than what I can't do."

Personalisation: "My pain is not my fault, and I will not blame myself for it. Instead, I will work towards finding ways to manage it and improve my quality of life."

Mind-reading: "I can't assume what others think about me. They might not understand my pain, but I can educate them and focus on my own journey towards healing."

Catastrophic thinking: "I will push myself within my limits and gradually increase my activity levels to manage my pain. With proper pacing and management, I can avoid worsening my pain.

Repeat the process:

Cognitive restructuring is an ongoing process, and it's important to continue identifying and challenging negative thoughts as they arise. Over time, this can change your beliefs about your pain and improve your ability to manage it.

In summary, cognitive restructuring involves identifying, evaluating, and challenging your negative thoughts and beliefs about pain and substituting them with more realistic and positive ones. This technique can be a powerful tool for managing chronic pain and improving overall well-being.

BEHAVIOUR MODIFICATION TECHNIQUES FOR CHRONIC PAIN MANAGEMENT

Behaviour modification is an essential component of cognitive-behavioural therapy (CBT). It is often used to help individuals manage chronic pain. Behaviour modification aims to help identify pain-related behaviours that may be contributing to pain and replace these behaviours with healthier ones.

- One example of behaviour modification is pacing. Pacing involves breaking up activities throughout the day into smaller, more feasible parts. By pacing, you can learn to avoid overexertion and prevent the pain from worsening.

- Another example is activity scheduling, which involves planning and scheduling enjoyable and meaningful activities into a daily routine. This can help to increase feelings of accomplishment, pleasure, and satisfaction, which can help to counteract negative thoughts and emotions associated with chronic pain.

- Deep breathing and progressive muscle relaxation are relaxation methods that can effectively alleviate muscle tension and induce relaxation. These techniques can help to reduce pain levels and improve overall well-being.

- Another behaviour modification strategy that may be useful is goal setting. Establishing goals can be a beneficial approach to concentrating on the activities you can do rather than those you cannot do. Goals need to be practical and attainable and should focus on activities that are important to you. Goals can help provide motivation, increase a sense of control and accomplishment, and improve overall well-being.

By identifying and changing pain-related behaviours, you can learn to manage the pain more effectively and improve your overall quality of life.

PRACTICAL TIPS

Here are some additional tips that may be useful for people with chronic pain to practice CBT.

- Keep a pain diary: Write down your pain levels, triggers, thoughts and feelings associated with your pain throughout the day. This can help you identify patterns, negative thoughts, and beliefs about pain that you may want to challenge with the help of CBT.

- Use positive affirmations: Create positive affirmations related to pain management, such as "I am capable of managing my pain" or "I can find ways to improve my quality of life despite my pain." Repeat these affirmations to yourself regularly to reinforce positive thinking.

- Practice relaxation techniques: Deep breathing, progressive muscle relaxation, guided imagery, and meditation are effective relaxation techniques that can help reduce stress, muscle tension, and pain.

- Mindfulness meditation: This practice involves concentrating on the present moment and acknowledging it without criticism. It can help reduce stress and anxiety related to chronic pain.

- Engage in pleasurable activities: Make time for enjoyable and fulfilling activities, even if they need to be modified to accommodate your pain. This can improve your mood and overall well-being.

- Gratitude practice: Focusing on what you are grateful for can shift the focus away from pain and negative thoughts. This practice can improve overall well-being and increase positivity.

- ◦ Surround yourself with supportive people: Create a supportive network by connecting with friends and family members who are empathetic and encouraging towards your pain management objectives. In addition, a support group or therapist with expertise in CBT for chronic pain can offer valuable assistance and direction.

CONCLUSION

CBT can be a helpful tool for managing chronic pain. It can help you to identify and challenge negative thoughts and beliefs about pain and to develop coping strategies for managing pain-related behaviours. Talk to your healthcare provider if you want to explore more about CBT as a treatment option for your chronic pain. Living well with chronic pain is possible with proper assistance and effective techniques.

12. Specialised Care for Chronic Pain

The Benefits and Role of Pain Clinics

INTRODUCTION

You may have been referred to a pain clinic if you have chronic pain. Pain clinics are specialist centres that focus on diagnosing and managing chronic pain. The goal of pain clinics is to help manage pain and improve the quality of life. This chapter will discuss the role of pain clinics in chronic pain.

WHAT IS A PAIN CLINIC?

A pain clinic is a specialised medical centre that provides comprehensive pain management services. Pain clinics are staffed by healthcare professionals specialising in treating chronic pain. These healthcare professionals may include pain specialists, physiotherapists, occupational therapists, psychologists, and nurses. Pain clinics may be located in hospitals or in the community.

REFERRAL PROCESS

Referral to a pain clinic can come from a primary care provider, a specialist, or a hospital. In some cases, patients may self-refer to a pain clinic.

WAIT TIMES

The wait time for an appointment at a pain clinic can vary depending on the clinic and the severity of the patient's condition. Sometimes, you may be able to get an appointment within a few weeks, while in other cases, the wait may be several months. Therefore, it's essential to ask the pain clinic about their wait times when making an appointment and to be prepared to wait for an opening if necessary. In some cases, pain clinics may have cancellation lists, which can help patients get an appointment sooner if an opening becomes available.

ROLE OF PAIN CLINICS IN CHRONIC PAIN MANAGEMENT

The primary role of pain clinics is to help patients manage their chronic pain. Pain clinics offer a holistic approach to managing pain by providing care from a group of healthcare providers collaborating to create a personalised treatment strategy for patients. This team approach allows pain clinics to address the many factors contributing to chronic pain, including physical, psychological, and social aspects.

TREATMENTS AVAILABLE IN PAIN CLINICS

Pain clinics provide an extensive array of therapies and interventions to manage chronic pain, including medication management, physical therapy, occupational therapy, psychological therapy, and interventional procedures. Medications used to treat chronic pain may include antidepressants and anticonvulsants. Physical and occupational therapy can help patients improve their physical functioning and reduce pain. Psychological therapy, such as cognitive-behavioural therapy (CBT), can help patients manage the emotional aspects of chronic pain. Interventional procedures like nerve blocks, infusions and injections into joints can provide pain relief for certain types of chronic pain.

It's crucial to remember that opioids may not always be the most suitable option for managing chronic pain. In fact, opioids may actually worsen chronic pain over time and lead to addiction and other serious health problems. Pain clinics recognise this and strive to provide their patients with safe and effective pain management options.

Certain pain clinics may provide specialised treatments, such as spinal cord stimulation and high-strength capsaicin patches (Qutenza), which are targeted for specific chronic pain conditions with localised neuropathic pain like Complex Regional Pain Syndrome (CRPS) and post-herpetic neuralgia respectively. If you are interested in these treatments, it is advisable to consult your healthcare provider. They can provide additional details and assess your eligibility for these interventions.

NERVE BLOCKS AND PAIN INTERVENTIONS

They are procedures that pain clinics may use to manage chronic pain. These procedures involve injecting medication, such as a local anaesthetic or steroid, close to a nerve to block pain signals. By numbing the affected nerves, these procedures can provide relief from pain.

Interventional procedures can be used to treat various chronic pain conditions, including joint pain, nerve pain, and spinal pain. The pain clinic team will use medical imaging, such as X-rays or ultrasound, to guide a needle or catheter to a specific body area. Once in place, medication can be injected directly into the affected area to relieve pain.

It is important to note that nerve blocks and pain interventions may not be appropriate or effective for all patients. The decision to use these treatments will depend on the type of chronic pain a patient is experiencing, their medical history and other individual factors. Additionally, there are potential risks and side effects associated with these procedures, which will be discussed with you before the procedure.

If you are considering nerve blocks or pain interventions, it is essential to discuss all treatment options with your healthcare provider and pain clinic team. You should also feel comfortable asking questions and expressing any concerns you may have about these procedures. The objective of the team at the pain clinic is to offer you optimal care and help you manage your chronic pain in a way that works best for your individual needs.

ROLE OF PAIN CLINICS IN PROVIDING EDUCATION AND SUPPORT FOR CHRONIC PAIN PATIENTS

In addition to providing treatment, pain clinics also offer education and support for you and your family. Pain clinics can provide information on pain management techniques, such as relaxation and mindfulness meditation. They can also offer advice on lifestyle changes to help patients manage their pain, such as exercise and healthy eating. Pain clinics can also provide support groups, which can be a valuable source of emotional support for patients with chronic pain.

WHO SHOULD CONSIDER GOING TO A PAIN CLINIC?

If chronic pain affects the quality of your life, you may benefit from going to a pain clinic. Pain clinics are typically recommended for patients with complex pain conditions that have not responded to other treatments. Pain clinics are also recommended for patients taking opioids for a long time and may benefit from a multidisciplinary approach to pain management.

HOW TO BENEFIT FROM ADVOCATING FOR YOURSELF AT A PAIN CLINIC

Advocating for yourself can be a vital part of managing chronic pain. It involves actively participating in your healthcare, asking questions, and working with your healthcare providers to formulate a personalised treatment plan that meets your needs. At a pain clinic, advocating for yourself can be especially important, as you will be working with a team of healthcare providers to manage your pain.

One way to advocate for yourself at a pain clinic is to be prepared for your appointments. Before your appointment, jot down any questions or concerns about your pain or treatment plan. In addition, make sure to have a complete and updated list of all the medications you are currently taking, including any over-the-counter drugs and dietary supplements, to bring to your appointment.

Another way to advocate for yourself is to be open and honest with your healthcare providers. Tell them about any changes in your pain, any adverse effects you are experiencing from your medications or any difficulties you are having with your treatment plan. Your healthcare providers are there to help you and need to know what is going on to give you the best possible care.

Finally, educating yourself about your condition and the treatments available for chronic pain can be helpful. This can assist you in asking knowledgeable questions and make informed decisions about your care. Your pain clinic can provide educational materials or refer you to reputable online resources.

Advocating for yourself can be a powerful tool in managing chronic pain. In addition, being an active participant in your healthcare can help ensure you receive the best possible care and treatment for your pain.

ADDITIONAL CONSIDERATIONS FOR CHRONIC PAIN PATIENTS

When considering whether to attend a pain clinic, a few additional factors may be essential to keep in mind. You can consider bringing a family member or friend to your appointment for emotional support and to help remember the necessary details discussed during your visit. Remembering that chronic pain management can be a long-term process, it's important to persist and be patient throughout the journey. However, with the support of a pain clinic team, many chronic pain patients can improve their quality of life and regain control over their pain.

CONCLUSION

Pain clinics play an essential role in the management of chronic pain. Pain clinics provide a multidisciplinary approach to pain management, which can help you manage your pain and improve your quality of life. If you have uncontrolled chronic pain, talk to your healthcare provider about whether a pain clinic may be right for you.

Step Four: Experiment with Coping Strategies

13. Coping with Flares and Exacerbations

Developing Resilience and Adaptability in the Face of Pain Fluctuations

INTRODUCTION

Living with chronic pain can be a complex and unpredictable journey. For many people, pain flares or exacerbations can occur suddenly and without warning, disrupting daily life and causing significant distress. Coping with these fluctuations requires a multifaceted approach that addresses both the physical and emotional impact of pain. In addition, developing resilience and adaptability in the face of pain fluctuations is critical to maintaining a sense of control and improving overall well-being.

This chapter will explore effective coping strategies for managing flares and exacerbations. We will look into how pain can manifest and discuss techniques for reducing pain, managing symptoms, and building resilience. By taking a comprehensive approach to managing flares, you can enhance your quality of life and regain control over your pain.

UNDERSTANDING FLARES AND EXACERBATIONS

Flares or exacerbations are an unfortunate reality for many individuals living with chronic pain. These periods are characterised by a sudden and significant increase in pain, as well as other symptoms like fatigue, sleep disturbances, and mood changes. Flares of pain can occur unexpectedly, significantly affecting an individual's day-to-day activities, making it difficult to perform even daily tasks or engage in social activities.

There are many potential triggers for flares, and these factors can differ from one individual to another. For example, stress is a common trigger for flares and can be caused by physical and emotional stressors. Changes in weather, such as changes in temperature or humidity, can also trigger flares for some individuals. Physical activity can be another trigger, particularly if the activity is new or involves a different type of movement than a person is used to.

It is essential for individuals with chronic pain to try to understand what triggers their flares so that they can develop effective coping strategies. By identifying the triggers, you may be able to modify your activities or lifestyle to reduce the frequency or intensity of flares. In addition, by understanding the triggers, you can better prepare for flares when they occur, allowing you to manage your symptoms more effectively.

MANAGING FLARES AND EXACERBATIONS

Multiple methods can be utilised to manage flares and exacerbations. The first step is to work with a healthcare provider to develop a plan for managing pain during flares. This may include medications, such as painkillers, and non-pharmacological approaches, such as heat or ice therapy, massage, or acupuncture.

In addition to these treatments, many self-care strategies can help manage flares. These include rest and relaxation techniques, such as deep breathing exercises or meditation, and gentle stretching or exercise programs, such as yoga or tai chi. It is essential to start slowly and gradually increase activity levels, as too much too soon can exacerbate pain and other symptoms.

BUILDING RESILIENCE

Coping with flares requires resilience and adaptability. Building resilience is a process of adapting and adjusting to the challenges of living with chronic pain. It is essential to recognise that flares are a natural part of living with chronic pain and develop coping strategies to help manage symptoms during these periods. Developing a positive outlook, staying connected with others, and participating in meaningful activities are vital to building resilience.

One way to build resilience is to practice positive thinking. This involves shifting the focus away from the negative aspects of living with chronic pain and instead focusing on the positive things in life. One approach for building resilience is to shift your focus towards your capabilities instead of limitations. For instance, you may choose to concentrate on the activities you can still perform rather than the ones you cannot. Positive thinking can help reduce stress, improve mood, and increase hope and optimism.

Maintaining social connections is also an important aspect of building resilience. Living with chronic pain can be a lonely experience, and having a support network of friends and family can offer emotional and practical assistance. In addition, connecting with a support group or an online community can offer a sense of belonging and understanding for individuals experiencing difficulties managing chronic pain.

Engaging in activities that bring joy and purpose is another way to build resilience. This may involve pursuing meaningful hobbies or interests, volunteering in the community, or taking on new challenges. Finding meaning and purpose in life can provide a sense of fulfilment and help manage the emotional impact of chronic pain.

Remember that developing resilience is a gradual process that requires time and effort. Coping with chronic pain can be difficult, but developing resilience can help individuals manage flares and exacerbations and maintain a positive outlook on life.

PRACTICE SELF-CARE

Self-care can be an essential tool in managing chronic flare-ups of pain in individuals with chronic pain because it helps you relax and recharge physically and emotionally. Flare-ups can be triggered by different factors, including physical and emotional stress, lack of sleep, poor diet, and overexertion. By practising self-care, individuals can proactively manage these triggers and reduce the severity and frequency of flare-ups. In addition, taking care of yourself can improve your mood, reduce stress, and help you feel more in control of your life.

There are many self-care activities that you can try, depending on your preferences and abilities. For example, one way to alleviate muscle and joint pain is to take a warm bath or shower, while practising yoga or meditation can reduce stress and promote relaxation. Participating in an enjoyable pastime, such as creating art or crafting, can provide a sense of achievement and diversion from the discomfort of chronic pain. Reading an enjoyable book or watching a favourite movie can also help to reduce stress and improve your mood.

It is beneficial to make self-care a regular part of your routine. This can be difficult, especially when dealing with chronic pain, but making time for self-care can help you feel better and improve your quality of life. You may need to experiment with different self-care activities to find what works best for you. However, once you find something you enjoy, try to integrate it into your everyday routine.

Remembering that self-care activities are not a luxury but a necessary part of managing chronic pain is essential. Taking time for yourself can help you to feel more energised and motivated to engage in other pain management strategies, such as physical therapy or medication management. So, make sure to prioritise self-care activities that you enjoy and that work for you and incorporate them into your daily routine.

CONCLUSION

Coping with flares and exacerbations requires a combination of strategies that aim to manage pain, reduce symptoms, and build resilience. Building resilience involves:

- Focusing on the positive aspects of life.
- Cultivating a positive mindset.
- Maintaining healthy social connections.
- Engaging in activities that bring meaning and joy.

It is a process that takes time and effort but can help individuals better cope with the challenges of living with chronic pain. By implementing these strategies, you can better manage the ups and downs of your condition and improve your overall quality of life.

14. Sleep Management for Chronic Pain

Improving Quality of Life and Pain Relief

INTRODUCTION

One of the most significant challenges for people with chronic pain is getting adequate sleep. Difficulty falling or staying asleep can be caused by pain, which can interfere with sleep. In addition, a lack of sleep can worsen the pain by increasing pain sensitivity. This vicious cycle can be frustrating and overwhelming for those who suffer from chronic pain.

Fortunately, there are some strategies which can help manage both pain and sleep problems. By understanding the relationship between pain and sleep and implementing some practical tips, it is possible to improve sleep quality and reduce the severity of pain. In this chapter, we will explore the connection between sleep and chronic pain and provide some strategies to help with pain management.

UNDERSTANDING SLEEP AND PAIN

Sleep is essential for physical and mental health. While sleeping, the body undergoes a restorative process where it repairs and rejuvenates tissues, and the brain integrates memories and regulates emotions. Unfortunately, pain can interfere with the quality and quantity of sleep, making it difficult to fall asleep, stay asleep, or get restorative sleep. Poor sleep can, in turn, worsen pain, creating a vicious cycle.

ANALOGY

Think of your body like a cellphone. Just like your phone needs to be charged to function correctly, your body needs sleep to repair and rejuvenate itself. Without enough sleep, your body can't heal and recover from chronic pain as effectively.

STRATEGIES FOR IMPROVING SLEEP

Improving sleep can help manage chronic pain. Here are some strategies to try:

- Establish a regular and consistent sleep routine by adhering to a regular bedtime and wake-up time every day. This helps regulate your body's internal clock, which improves your sleep.

- Create a sleep-friendly environment: Ensure your bedroom is cool, quiet, and dark.

- Create a calming bedtime ritual, such as soaking in a warm bath, reading a book, or engaging in relaxation exercises like deep breathing or progressive muscle relaxation.

- Consider using a comfortable mattress and pillow that provide proper support and alignment for your body.

- Try relaxation techniques like aromatherapy, calming music, or white noise machines to create a peaceful sleep environment.

- Avoid caffeine and alcohol, particularly in the evenings. Caffeine is a stimulant which can make it difficult to fall asleep, while alcohol can interfere with the quality of your sleep. In addition, these substances can interfere with sleep and worsen pain.

- Avoid large meals, and heavy or spicy foods before bedtime.

- Practice good sleep hygiene by avoiding stimulating activities like watching TV or using electronic devices in bed.

- Exercise regularly: This can help improve your sleep quality and reduce pain.
- Avoid daytime naps: Daytime napping can interfere with nighttime sleep.
- Manage pain before bedtime: Take pain medications as prescribed.
- Practice relaxation techniques before bed to calm your mind and prepare for sleep. This can include deep breathing, meditation, or gentle stretching.
- Consider incorporating gentle exercise, such as yoga or stretching, into your daily routine. Exercise can help reduce pain and improve sleep quality.
- Consider cognitive behavioural therapy for insomnia (CBT-I) or other psychological treatments to address underlying psychological factors affecting your sleep.
- Use pain management techniques, such as hot or cold compresses or transcutaneous electrical nerve stimulation (TENS), to reduce pain before bedtime.
- Consider using over-the-counter sleep aids or prescription medications, but only under the guidance of a healthcare provider.
- Keep a sleep diary to track and record your sleep patterns and identify any triggers that may affect your sleep.
- Consider discussing your sleep issues with your healthcare provider without hesitation. They can identify if there are any underlying conditions, such as sleep apnea, that may contribute to your sleep problems and recommend any treatment if required.

Remember that good sleep hygiene is a crucial component of chronic pain management. By prioritising restful, restorative sleep, you can help reduce pain and improve your overall quality of life.

CONCLUSION

Sleep problems can worsen chronic pain, and chronic pain can interfere with sleep. By understanding the connection between sleep and pain and implementing strategies to improve sleep, individuals with chronic pain can improve their overall health and quality of life.

15. Mood and Chronic Pain

Strategies to Help with Pain

INTRODUCTION

Living with persistent pain can be a difficult and tiring ordeal, significantly impacting an individual's mood and mental health. Chronic pain often goes hand-in-hand with feelings of depression, anxiety, and stress, which can exacerbate pain and make it more challenging to manage. Despite the challenges and exhaustion of living with chronic pain, various strategies can be implemented to improve mood and reduce pain. This chapter will explore the connection between mood and chronic pain and provide practical tips for managing both.

UNDERSTANDING THE CONNECTION BETWEEN MOOD AND CHRONIC PAIN

Chronic pain can significantly impact an individual's mental health and mood. The persistent experience of pain can lead to feelings of frustration, anger, and hopelessness, making it challenging to engage in everyday activities. The emotional impact of chronic pain can also exacerbate the physical symptoms, creating a vicious cycle of pain and negative emotions.

Furthermore, depression, anxiety, and stress can all contribute to the experience of chronic pain. People who have chronic pain are at a higher risk of experiencing symptoms of depression and anxiety, and these conditions can worsen the pain. For example, anxiety can heighten sensitivity to pain and cause individuals to perceive pain as more intense than it actually is.

ANALOGIES

Here are some analogies to describe the relationship between mood and chronic pain:

Imagine a jar filled with marbles. Each marble represents a thought or emotion. When the jar becomes too full, the marbles spill out and create chaos. Similarly, when our minds become too full of negative thoughts and feelings, they can spill out and worsen our experience of chronic pain.

Chronic pain can be like a storm cloud that follows you everywhere. Seeing any light or positivity in your life can be challenging when the cloud is dark and heavy. Taking steps to improve your mood can help to dissipate the storm cloud and create a more positive outlook.

Chronic pain can be like a heavy backpack you carry all the time. Negative emotions can make the backpack feel even heavier, while positive emotions can make it feel lighter and more manageable.

Remember that chronic pain and mood are closely linked, and improving one can positively impact the other. Individuals with chronic pain can experience a better quality of life by implementing strategies to improve their mood.

STRATEGIES FOR IMPROVING MOOD AND REDUCING PAIN

Here are some techniques which can help improve mood and reduce pain:

- Engage in enjoyable activities: Participating in enjoyable activities can help boost mood and reduce pain. Try to participate in pleasurable activities, spend quality time with family and friends, and find new interests and hobbies.

- Practising relaxation techniques like deep breathing and meditation can reduce your stress and anxiety, reducing pain.

- Practice mindfulness to help manage negative thoughts and emotions. One can practice mindfulness by focusing on the present moment and refraining from evaluative thoughts. This can be done through meditation or taking a few deep breaths and concentrating on the sensation of the breath.

- Cognitive-behavioural therapy: Cognitive-behavioural therapy (CBT) is a form of treatment that helps individuals identify and change negative thoughts and behaviours contributing to pain and mood disturbances.

- Exercise regularly: Regular exercise can help improve mood and reduce pain. Low-impact exercises, like walking, swimming, and yoga, can benefit individuals with chronic pain.

- Getting adequate sleep is crucial for maintaining both physical and mental health. Getting enough restorative sleep can help improve mood and reduce pain.

- Eating a balanced diet can help improve mood and decrease inflammation, which can contribute to pain.

- Seek support: Living with chronic pain can be challenging, and seeking support from loved ones and healthcare providers is essential.

CONCLUSION

Chronic pain can significantly affect mental and emotional well-being, and mood and mental health can affect pain. By understanding the connection between mood and pain and implementing strategies to improve both, individuals with chronic pain can improve their overall health and quality of life. Discuss with your healthcare provider if you continue to have difficulty managing pain or improving your mood, as there may be underlying conditions that require treatment.

16. Effective Activity Pacing

Understanding the importance of Pacing for Chronic Pain Management

INTRODUCTION

If you experience chronic pain, you know it can be challenging to balance your desire to stay active with the need to avoid exacerbating your symptoms. Pacing your activities is a demonstrated approach that can aid in managing pain and enhancing your ability to participate in significant activities. In this chapter, I will explain pacing and why it is essential and provide practical tips and exercises to help you incorporate pacing into your daily routine.

WHAT IS PACING?

Pacing is a strategy that involves breaking up activities into manageable chunks to avoid overexertion and minimise the risk of pain flare-ups. By pacing your activities, you can conserve energy and reduce the physical and emotional toll of chronic pain.

WHY IS PACING IMPORTANT?

Pacing is essential for several reasons.

- First, it allows you to avoid overexertion, which can exacerbate your symptoms and increase pain and fatigue.
- Second, pacing helps you build endurance over time, enabling you to gradually increase your activity level without triggering pain flare-ups.

○ Third, pacing can help you stay engaged in meaningful activities, essential for maintaining a positive outlook and overall well-being.

ANALOGIES

Think of pacing like a marathon race. You wouldn't start sprinting at the beginning and exhaust yourself before the finish line. Instead, you pace yourself, conserving energy so that you can make it to the end. Similarly, pacing your activities can help you preserve energy and manage your pain throughout the day.

Pacing can be compared to driving a car with limited fuel. For instance, just as you would not accelerate quickly or brake suddenly to save fuel, you should not overexert yourself with activities that may exacerbate your pain. Instead, you drive steadily and smoothly, avoiding sharp movements to ensure that you get the most out of your fuel. Similarly, pacing your activities can help you manage your energy and avoid exacerbating your pain.

Pacing can be thought of as cooking a meal on low heat. You wouldn't turn up the heat to maximum and burn the meal because you want to eat it as soon as possible. Instead, you cook it slowly and steadily so it turns out perfectly. Similarly, pacing your activities can help you manage your pain and achieve your goals over time without burning out or causing flare-ups.

INDIVIDUALISED PAIN MANAGEMENT PLAN - COMBINING PACING AND OTHER STRATEGIES

It's important to note that pacing activities may only work for some and may take time to find the right balance which works for you. Additionally, it's crucial to develop an individualised pain management plan that incorporates pacing and other strategies. Finally, you can improve your overall well-being and quality of life by taking a comprehensive approach to managing chronic pain, including physical therapy, medication, and self-care.

TIPS FOR PACING ACTIVITIES

- Set Realistic Goals: When pacing activities, it's essential to set realistic goals that consider your current level of functioning. Start by breaking down tasks into smaller, more manageable steps, and gradually increase the length and intensity of your activities over time.

- Plan Ahead: Before starting an activity, please take a moment to plan out how you will approach it. Consider factors such as how long the activity will take, how much energy it will require, and whether you need to take breaks. By planning ahead, you can pace yourself more effectively and reduce the risk of pain flare-ups.

- Monitor Your Symptoms: Pay close attention to your symptoms during and after activities. For example, if you observe a rise in pain or other indications, it could indicate that you should alter your pacing or take a break.

- Use Adaptive Strategies: Adaptive strategies, such as using assistive devices or modifying your environment, can help conserve energy and reduce pain during activities. For example, using a rolling cart to transport heavy items or sitting on a stool while cooking can help you avoid overexertion.

- Start Small: Choose an activity you enjoy, and practice pacing it over the course of a week. Start by breaking the activity into smaller chunks, for example, 10 minutes at a time, and gradually increase the length of each session over time.

- Practice Mindful Movement: Mindful movements, such as gentle yoga or tai chi, can help you improve your body awareness and pacing skills. Start with simple activities, such as seated stretches, and gradually build up to more challenging postures.

- Use a Timer: Using a timer can help you stay on track and

avoid overexertion. Set a timer for each activity or task, and take breaks as needed to rest and recharge.

CONCLUSION

Pacing activities is a valuable strategy for managing chronic pain and improving your quality of life. By setting realistic goals, planning, monitoring your symptoms, and using adaptive strategies, you can conserve energy and reduce the physical and emotional toll of chronic pain. In addition, with practice and perseverance, pacing can help you stay engaged in meaningful activities and achieve your goals. Finally, it is crucial to remember that pacing activities should not be utilised to completely avoid physical activity but instead as a technique to handle symptoms and participate in meaningful activities.

17. Somatic Exercises to Ease Chronic Pain

Unleashing Body Wisdom

INTRODUCTION

Living with chronic pain presents many challenges, both physical and emotional. In addition to medical interventions, incorporating somatic exercises into your pain management toolbox can significantly enhance your coping strategies. This chapter explores the benefits of somatic exercises and provides practical guidance on integrating them into your daily routine.

UNDERSTANDING SOMATIC EXERCISES

Somatic exercises focus on re-educating the body's movement patterns and increasing body awareness. By bringing attention to your body and engaging in gentle, mindful movements, somatic exercises can help you develop a stronger connection with your body and gain greater control over your pain. In addition, these exercises focus on releasing tension, improving mobility, and promoting relaxation, all contributing to reducing pain and discomfort. Through the practice of somatic exercises, you can learn to listen to your body's signals, find areas of tension or imbalance, and respond with gentle movements and conscious breathwork. This process of self-awareness and self-care allows you to actively participate in your pain management journey, empowering you to find relief and improve your overall well-being. With regular practice, somatic exercises can help you cultivate resilience, improve your pain-coping strategies, and enhance your quality of life.

BODY-MIND INTEGRATION

Chronic pain often disrupts the natural harmony between the mind and body. Somatic exercises help re-establish this connection by emphasising mindful movement and body awareness. In addition, by intentionally tuning into the body's signals and sensations during workouts, you develop a deeper understanding of how pain manifests and how it can be managed.

SOMATIC EXERCISE TECHNIQUES FOR COPING WITH CHRONIC PAIN

Pandiculation:

Pandiculation is a core technique used in somatic exercises. It involves contracting and releasing muscles to reset their resting length and improve muscle coordination. By consciously pandiculating various muscle groups, you can release chronic muscle tension, improve your range of motion, and alleviate pain. In addition, incorporating gentle pandiculation exercises into your daily routine can significantly enhance your coping strategies.

Slow and Mindful Movements:

Engaging in slow, deliberate movements with mindful awareness can help unravel patterns of tension and discomfort associated with chronic pain. This includes gentle stretching, rotations, and movements that target specific areas of pain or stiffness. By moving slowly and paying particular attention to the sensations that arise, you can find areas of restriction and explore pain-free ranges of motion.

Progressive Relaxation Techniques:

Progressive relaxation techniques involve systematically tensing and releasing different muscle groups to promote relaxation and reduce muscular tension. By focusing on specific areas of pain or tightness and progressively relaxing them, you can enhance your body's natural relaxation response and experience relief from chronic pain.

Mind-Body Integration Practices:

Combining somatic exercises with other mind-body practices, such as meditation or mindfulness, amplifies their effectiveness. These practices foster a more profound sense of relaxation, cultivate a compassionate attitude toward yourself and your pain, and strengthen your overall coping strategies. Incorporating these practices into your routine creates a comprehensive approach to managing chronic pain.

BENEFITS OF SOMATIC EXERCISES FOR COPING WITH CHRONIC PAIN

- Increased Body Awareness: Somatic exercises improve your ability to listen to your body's signals and respond appropriately. This heightened body awareness enables you to find and address areas of tension or discomfort, promoting self-care and pain management.

- Relaxation and Stress Reduction: Somatic exercises elicit a relaxation response, reducing stress levels and promoting a sense of calm. By following these exercises, you can effectively manage the physical and emotional stress associated with chronic pain.

- Improved Muscle Function: Somatic exercises retrain your muscles to move efficiently and restore proper alignment.

BREATHWORK AND BODY AWARENESS

Integrating breathwork into somatic exercises enhances body awareness and relaxation. By synchronising your breathing with movements, you can facilitate the release of tension. As a result, you can significantly improve their effectiveness in managing chronic pain. Breathwork techniques, such as deep breathing, diaphragmatic breathing, or mindful breathing, bring attention and intention to the breath, promoting relaxation, body awareness, and a sense of calm. By consciously coordinating the breath with specific movements and stretches during somatic exercises, individuals can deepen their mind-body connection and enhance the overall therapeutic benefits. It helps create a harmonious rhythm between the body and mind, facilitating a sense of balance, stability, and inner peace.

ANALOGY

Imagine you are a sculptor working with a block of clay. The clay represents your body, and chronic pain is like a hardened knot within it. As you engage in somatic exercises and integrate breathwork, it's as if you're applying gentle pressure and adding water to the clay, gradually softening and loosening the hardened knot. With each breath and movement, you're able to reshape and mould the clay, untangling the knot and allowing the pain to dissipate.

Just as a sculptor uses their hands and tools to transform the clay, you use somatic exercises and breathwork to transform your body. By cultivating body awareness, you become attuned to the subtle sensations and signals within, much like a sculptor who feels the texture and malleability of the clay. The breath becomes your guiding force, providing the necessary flow and rhythm to unravel the knot of pain.

You are untangling the knot with each conscious breath and movement, finding liberation and relief. Just as the sculptor sees the clay taking shape and form, you experience your body becoming more flexible, relaxed, and free from pain. It's a gradual and mindful process requiring patience and gentle persistence. Still, with each session of somatic exercises and breathwork, you're sculpting a new relationship with your body and discovering its innate capacity for healing.

In this analogy, you are the artist of your own body, using somatic exercises and breathwork as your tools to transform pain into freedom. Embrace this creative process and allow yourself to discover the profound healing power of consciously untangling the knot of chronic pain.

STEPS FOR SOME EASY SOMATIC EXERCISES

Here are some somatic exercises that integrate breathwork. It is important to adjust the exercises according to your comfort level. Respecting your limits and not pushing yourself beyond what feels safe and manageable is essential. If you encounter any sensations of pain or discomfort while performing the exercises, modify or discontinue them as needed. Remember, the goal is to support your well-being and manage chronic pain, so prioritise self-care and take it at your own pace. Regular practice of these breath-integrated somatic exercises can be valuable in managing and coping with chronic pain.

NECK

Gentle Head Tilts:

- Assume a position that feels comfortable for you, whether sitting or standing, and make sure to maintain proper posture.
- Let your shoulders relax and allow your arms to naturally rest at your sides in a comfortable manner.
- Inhale deeply and exhale gradually to promote relaxation throughout your body.
- Gently tilt your head to the right side, bringing your right ear closer to your right shoulder.
- Hold the tilted position for a few seconds, feeling a gentle stretch on the left side of your neck.
- Return your head to the neutral position.
- Perform the same tilt on the opposite side, bringing your left ear closer to your left shoulder once again.
- Maintain the position briefly before returning to the neutral starting position.
- Repeat the exercise 3-5 times on each side, moving slowly without strain.

Neck Rotations:

- Start in a comfortable seated or standing position with good posture.
- Let your shoulders relax and allow your arms to naturally rest at your sides in a comfortable manner.
- Inhale deeply and exhale gradually to promote relaxation throughout your body.
- Gently turn your head to the right side as if you're looking over your right shoulder.
- Pause for a moment, feeling a gentle stretch along the left side of your neck.
- Return your head to the centre, facing forward.
- Repeat the rotation to the left side, looking over your left shoulder.
- Pause and return to the centre.
- Repeat the exercise 3-5 times on each side, moving slowly and smoothly.

Neck Stretches:

- Assume a sitting or standing position that feels comfortable to you while maintaining good posture.
- Let your shoulders relax and allow your arms to naturally rest at your sides comfortably.
- Inhale deeply and exhale gradually to promote relaxation throughout your body.
- Slowly lower your head, tilting it forward to bring your chin closer to your chest.
- Experience a mild stretching sensation along the posterior side of your neck.
- Hold the stretch for a few seconds.
- Return your head to the neutral position.
- Next, tilt your head backwards, looking up toward the ceiling.
- Experience a subtle stretching sensation at the front of your neck.

- Hold the stretch briefly.
- Return your head to neutral.
- Repeat the sequence 3-5 times, moving slowly and smoothly.

SHOULDER

Shoulder Roll and Release:

- Begin by assuming a relaxed and comfortable seated or standing position.
- Keep your arms relaxed at your sides.
- Take a moment to tune into your body and bring awareness to your shoulders.
- Slowly inhale deeply, and as you release the breath, softly raise your shoulders towards your ears, then move them in a circular motion, gradually rolling them back and down, squeezing your shoulder blades together as they move down and back.
- Repeat this shoulder roll movement several times, allowing your shoulders to move in a smooth and controlled manner.
- As you roll your shoulders, pay attention to any areas of tension or discomfort. When you encounter a tense spot, pause and take a deep breath, consciously releasing any tension in that area.
- Continue the shoulder roll, focusing on gradually relaxing and releasing any tightness or pain in your shoulders.
- After a few rounds of shoulder rolls, take a moment to notice any changes in the sensation and mobility of your shoulders.

Gentle Stretches for the Shoulder Muscles:

- Stand or sit comfortably with good posture.
- Relax your arms by your sides.
- Inhale deeply, allowing your breath to fill your lungs and consciously relaxing your body.
- Slowly raise one arm in front of you until it is parallel to

the ground.

- Gently reach across your chest with the raised arm, using your other hand to support and guide the stretch.
- Experience a mild stretching sensation in the posterior region of your shoulder.
- Hold the stretch for 15-30 seconds while breathing deeply.
- Relax the stretch and then repeat the movement on the opposite side.
- Perform the stretch 2-3 times on each side, alternating between sides.

BACK

Arching and Rounding the Back:

- Assume a comfortable seated or standing position, ensuring proper posture.
- Relax your arms by your sides.
- Inhale deeply, allowing your breath to fill your lungs and promote relaxation throughout your body.
- Slowly and gently arch your back, pushing your chest forward and allowing your shoulder blades to come closer together.
- Maintain the arched position for a few moments, experiencing a subtle stretching sensation along the anterior part of your body.
- Return to the neutral position.
- Proceed by gradually rounding your back, gently moving your shoulders forward and drawing your chin closer to your chest.
- Hold the rounded position for a few seconds, feeling a gentle stretch along the back of your body.
- Return to the neutral position.
- Repeat the sequence 3-5 times, moving slowly and smoothly.

Spinal Twists:

- Position yourself at the edge of a chair or on the floor,

comfortably crossing your legs.
- Position your right hand on your left knee or thigh, finding a comfortable placement.
- Inhale deeply, lengthening your spine.
- As you exhale, softly rotate your upper body towards the left, allowing your right hand to guide the movement.
- Ensure that your head remains in alignment with your spine, avoiding any excessive strain or tension in your neck.
- Hold the twist for a few breaths, feeling a gentle stretch along your back.
- Inhale to unwind and return to the starting position.
- Repeat the twisting movement to the opposite side, this time placing your left hand on your right knee or thigh.
- Perform the sequence 2-3 times on each side, moving slowly without strain.

Gentle Backbends:
- Assume a standing position with your feet positioned hip-width apart, or alternatively, sit on the edge of a chair with your back maintaining a straight posture.
- Position your hands on your lower back, with your fingers pointing downward.
- Inhale deeply, lengthening your spine.
- Exhale as you gently lean back, arching your upper back and opening your chest.
- Keep your neck relaxed and avoid straining your neck.
- Maintain the backbend position for a few breaths, allowing yourself to experience a gentle stretching sensation along the front of your body.
- Inhale to return to an upright position.
- Repeat the backbend 3-5 times, moving slowly and smoothly.

HIP

Hip Circles:

- Assume a standing position with your feet positioned hip-width apart or sit on the edge of a chair while maintaining good posture.
- Relax your arms by your sides.
- Inhale deeply, allowing your breath to deeply relax your entire body.
- Slowly and gently circle your hips in a circular motion.
- Start by moving your hips forward, then to the right, back, and to the left, completing a full circle.
- Move smoothly and with control, feeling the movement in your hip joints.
- After a few circles in one direction, reverse the direction and circle your hips in the opposite direction.
- Repeat the exercise 3-5 times in each direction, moving slowly and smoothly.

Gentle Stretches for the Hip Flexors and Gluteal Muscles:

- Assume a lunge position by stepping your right leg forward and extending your left leg behind you.
- Maintain an upright position with your torso and keep your back straight throughout the exercise.
- Gradually and carefully lower your left knee towards the ground, allowing a gentle stretch to be felt in the front area of your left hip.
- Place your hands on your right thigh for support and balance.
- Hold the stretch for 15-30 seconds while breathing deeply.
- Relax the stretch and proceed to repeat the same sequence on the other side, with your left leg positioned forward and your right leg extended behind you.
- Perform the stretch 2-3 times on each side, alternating between sides.

Supine Hip Opening:

- Recline on your back, finding a comfortable surface such as a yoga mat or a padded area.

- Close your eyes, gently take a few deep breaths and allow your body to relax.
- Let your mind focus on the present moment.
- Bring your attention to your hips and notice any sensations or discomfort in that area.
- As you inhale, imagine your breath flowing into your hips, bringing a sense of relaxation and release.
- As you exhale, gently draw one knee towards your chest, using your hands to support the movement if needed.
- Inhale deeply, and as you exhale, slowly and mindfully lower the knee to the side, aiming to bring it towards the floor.
- As you lower the knee, visualize any tension or pain in your hip melting away with each breath out.
- Please take a moment to observe the sensations in your hip as it opens and notice any changes in comfort or discomfort.
- Inhale again, drawing the breath into your body, and slowly bring the knee back to the starting position as you exhale.
- Repeat the movement with the other leg, gently drawing the knee towards your chest and then lowering it to the side.
- Continue alternating between legs, moving at a comfortable and gentle pace.
- Throughout the exercise, maintain a steady and relaxed breath, using each breath to soften and relax the hip area.
- Only move the leg as far as feels comfortable for you.
- Complete several repetitions on each side, and slowly bring the movement to a close when you're ready.

KNEE

Knee Circles:

- Assume a standing position with your feet positioned hip-width apart or sit on the edge of a chair while maintaining proper posture.

- Relax your arms by your sides.
- Inhale deeply, allowing your breath to fill your lungs and promote a state of relaxation in your body.
- Raise your right foot slightly off the ground while maintaining a bent knee position.
- Slowly and gently rotate your right knee in a circular motion.
- Move the knee to the right, forward, to the left, and back to complete a full circle.
- Keep the movements smooth and controlled, feeling the rotation in your knee joint.
- After a few circles in one direction, reverse the direction and circle your knee in the opposite direction.
- Repeat the exercise 3-5 times in each direction, then switch to your left knee and repeat.

Gentle Knee Bends:

- Assume a standing position with your feet positioned hip-width apart or sit on the edge of a chair while maintaining proper posture.
- Relax your arms by your sides.
- Inhale deeply, allowing your breath to flow into your body and promote a sense of relaxation throughout.
- Gradually and softly bend your knees, descending your body as if you were settling into a seated position on an imaginary chair.
- Maintain contact between your heels and the ground while ensuring proper alignment by keeping your knees aligned with your toes during the exercise.
- Pause in the bent position for a few seconds, feeling the stretch in your thighs and glutes.
- Slowly straighten your knees and return to an upright position.
- Repeat the knee bends 8-10 times, moving slowly and smoothly.

Knee Extensions:

- Position yourself at the front edge of a chair, maintaining proper posture.
- Position your feet flat on the ground, positioned hip-width apart, with the soles of your feet fully touching the ground.
- Inhale deeply, allowing your breath to fill your lungs and promote a sense of relaxation throughout your body.
- Gradually and gently extend one leg forward, straightening the knee to a comfortable extent.
- Maintain the extended position for a few moments, experiencing a mild stretching sensation in the back of your thigh.
- Slowly bend your knee and return your foot to the ground.
- Repeat the knee extension with the other leg.
- Perform the exercise 8-10 times on each leg, alternating between legs.

ANKLE

Ankle Circles:

- Begin by assuming a relaxed and comfortable seated or standing position.
- Maintain the position with your legs extended straight in front of you.
- Begin by slowly circling your ankle clockwise, making gentle and controlled movements.
- As you circle your ankle, focus on bringing awareness to your ankle and foot sensations.
- Pay attention to any areas of tension, discomfort, or restricted movement.
- Take slow, deep breaths and imagine the breath flowing into your ankle, helping to release tension and promote relaxation.
- After a few circles in one direction, switch to circling your ankle counterclockwise.

- Continue circling your ankle in both directions for several rounds, allowing your ankle to move freely and comfortably.
- If you encounter any areas of tightness or pain, pause, breathe deeply, and visualize the tension melting away.
- After completing the ankle circles, take a moment to notice any changes in the sensation and mobility of your ankle.
- Remember to perform this exercise within a pain-free range of motion and modify it to suit your comfort level.

FOOT

Toe Curls:

- Settle yourself on a chair or find a seated position that feels comfortable to you.
- Place your feet flat on the ground.
- Start with your right foot and curl your toes inward as if gripping the ground.
- Hold the curled position for a few seconds, then release and relax your toes.
- Repeat the toe curls with your left foot.
- Perform the exercise 8-10 times on each foot.

Foot Stretches:

- Sit on a chair or find a seated position where you feel comfortable and supported.
- Slowly and gently straighten your right leg forward, keeping your heel grounded throughout the movement.
- Flex your right foot, pointing your toes toward your knee.
- Hold the stretch for a few seconds, feeling a gentle stretch along the top of your foot.
- Release the stretch and relax your foot.
- Next, extend your right leg again, and this time, point your toes away from your knee, stretching the bottom of your foot.

- Maintain the stretched position for a few seconds, allowing the muscles to gently elongate and relax, then release and bring your right leg back to the starting position.
- Repeat the stretches with your left foot.
- Perform the stretches 2-3 times on each foot.

ELBOW

Elbow Bends:

- Sit on a chair or stand with good posture.
- Relax your arms by your sides.
- Inhale deeply, allowing your breath to flow into your body, promoting relaxation throughout your entire body.
- Slowly and gently bend your elbows, bringing your hands towards your shoulders.
- Ensure that your upper arms remain still and positioned close to your sides throughout the exercise.
- Pause in the bent position for a few seconds, feeling the stretch in the muscles around your elbows.
- Gradually extend your elbows, straightening your arms, and then return the elbow gently to the starting position in a slow and controlled manner.
- Repeat the elbow bends 8-10 times, moving slowly and smoothly.

Forearm Rotations:

- Sit on a chair or stand with good posture.
- Relax your arms by your sides.
- Inhale deeply, allowing your breath to fill your lungs and promote a sense of relaxation throughout your body.
- Extend your arms forward, keeping them parallel to the ground, with your palms facing downward.
- Slowly rotate your forearms in a circular motion, moving from the elbows.
- Rotate your hands to face upwards, then return until your palms face down again.

- Feel the movement and stretch in your forearms.
- Repeat the exercise 5-8 times.

WRIST

Wrist Flexion and Extension:

- Sit on a chair or stand with good posture.
- Relax your arms by your sides.
- Inhale deeply, allowing your breath to flow into your body and promote a sense of relaxation throughout.
- Stretch your arms forward, positioning them parallel to the ground, with your palms facing downwards.
- Slowly and gently flex your wrists, bringing your fingertips toward your forearms.
- Hold the flexed position for a few seconds, feeling the stretch in the top of your forearms and wrists.
- Return your wrists to the neutral position.
- Next, slowly and gently extend your wrists, moving your fingertips away from your forearms.
- Keep the extended position for a few seconds, experiencing a stretching sensation in the underside of your forearms and wrists.
- Return your wrists to the neutral position.
- Repeat the flexion and extension movements 8-10 times, moving slowly and smoothly.

APPROACHING SOMATIC EXERCISES SAFELY AND EFFECTIVELY FOR CHRONIC PAIN MANAGEMENT

Engaging in somatic exercises can be helpful for individuals with chronic pain, even if they find normal daily activities painful. It's understandable to be cautious about trying new exercises when there is a fear of exacerbating pain. However, somatic exercises are specifically designed to promote relaxation, release muscle tension, and improve body awareness, which can ultimately help manage chronic pain.

To approach these exercises safely and confidently, starting gently and gradually increasing the intensity as tolerated is essential. Begin with simple movements and progress at your own pace. Listening to your body is crucial throughout the process; if an exercise causes excessive pain, modifying or choosing an alternative exercise is recommended. Consulting with a healthcare professional or a qualified somatic movement practitioner can provide guidance tailored to your specific needs. Remember, the goal is not to push through the pain but to establish a gentle and mindful movement practice that can bring relief and improved well-being over time.

CONCLUSION

Through the practice of somatic therapy, we can unlock the potential for healing and coping with chronic pain. By nurturing the mind-body connection, engaging in practical techniques, and embracing movement and visualisation, you can experience relief, reduce pain, and reclaim control over your life. Remember, each person's journey is unique, so explore and adapt these techniques to suit your specific needs and preferences. It is essential to understand that somatic intelligence is an ongoing process of self-discovery to empower your pain management.

Step Five: Build a Support System

18. *Building a Support System*

The Importance of Social Support and Advocacy in Coping with Chronic Pain

INTRODUCTION

Chronic pain is a complex and pervasive issue affecting millions worldwide. This chapter will discuss the critical role that social support and advocacy can play in helping individuals cope with chronic pain. This chapter will also explore the various types of support that can be helpful, including emotional support from loved ones, practical support in managing daily activities, and informational support from healthcare professionals and online resources.

By providing practical tips and advice for seeking out and cultivating supportive relationships and resources, I hope to empower readers to take an active role in managing their chronic pain and improving their quality of life.

WHAT IS A SUPPORT SYSTEM?

A support system refers to a group of individuals and resources that provide emotional, practical, and medical support to help you cope with chronic pain. Your support system may include family, friends, healthcare providers, support groups, and community resources. A staunch support system can help you feel less alone, provide encouragement and motivation, and offer practical help with tasks which may be difficult or impossible to do on your own.

ANALOGY

Building a support system is like building a safety net. Just as a safety net catches you if you fall, a support system catches you when you need help. Your support system can provide emotional, practical, and social support to help you navigate the challenges of chronic pain. Feel free to reach out to your support network when you need help.

IMPORTANCE OF A SUPPORT SYSTEM

Social support can help people with chronic pain in various ways. It can provide emotional support, which can be essential for managing the psychological impact of chronic pain. Chronic pain can lead to feelings of anxiety, depression, and social isolation. It can be highly advantageous to have a person who can empathise with your situation and provide a listening ear. When you need to vent or talk about your struggles, emotional support can come from friends and family members who offer empathy, understanding, and a listening ear. Emotional support can help you stay motivated and optimistic, even on difficult days.

Social support can provide informational support, which can be especially helpful when navigating the healthcare system. In addition, support from healthcare professionals and peers with chronic pain experience can help you access information and resources about treatment options, pain management strategies, and coping techniques.

Practical support, such as help with daily tasks like cooking, cleaning, or grocery shopping, can be invaluable for people with chronic pain. Living with chronic pain can make even simple tasks difficult or impossible. Practical support from friends, family, or community resources can help ease the burden and allow you to focus on your recovery.

Medical support can come from healthcare providers who offer pain management strategies and treatment options.

A support system can also provide a sense of belonging, which can be especially important for those with chronic pain who may feel isolated or disconnected. Support groups, either in-person or online, can provide an opportunity to meet others who are going through the same challenges and offer a space for sharing advice, resources, and coping strategies.

Ultimately, a support system can help you feel empowered and more in control of your life as you manage your chronic pain and advocate for your needs. In addition, individuals with chronic pain with a solid social support network tend to have improved physical and mental health outcomes compared to those without such support.

ANALOGY

Social support is like a warm blanket. Social support can help reduce stress and anxiety and improve your mood and outlook on life. Think of social support like a warm blanket on a cold day - it provides comfort and security when you need it most.

BUILDING A SUPPORT NETWORK

Creating a support system is crucial in the management of chronic pain. When dealing with chronic pain, it is common to feel alone and isolated. But having a support network can make all the difference in how you cope with pain. Therefore, reaching out to people who can provide emotional support and help you navigate the challenges of living with chronic pain is essential.

People close to you, such as friends and family, can provide valuable support when managing chronic pain. They can provide emotional support, help with daily tasks, and offer a listening ear when you need to talk. It's essential to communicate with your loved ones about your pain and how it affects your life, so they can understand your needs and provide the support you need.

People with chronic pain can benefit from joining support groups offering emotional support, guidance, and advice from others experiencing similar challenges. These groups can provide a sense of community and understanding and offer a safe space to share your experiences and learn from others. Support groups can provide helpful assistance for those living with chronic pain. Whether in-person or online, these groups provide opportunities to meet and communicate with people with similar difficulties and access information and advice on managing pain.

In addition to friends, family, and support groups, healthcare professionals can also be part of your support network. Your healthcare provider can provide medical treatment for your pain and advise on managing your symptoms. They can also refer you to other healthcare professionals, such as physical therapists, occupational therapists, or mental health professionals, who can assist in managing pain and enhancing one's overall quality of life.

Building a support network takes time and effort, but it can be crucial to managing chronic pain. It would be best to remember that support is available to you and that you are not alone in dealing with chronic pain.

ADVOCACY AND SELF-ADVOCACY

Advocacy is another essential part of building a support system for people with chronic pain. It means speaking up for yourself and your needs and working to promote your rights and access to resources that can help manage your pain. This can involve seeking healthcare providers knowledgeable about chronic pain and advocating for policy changes to improve access to pain management resources.

Self-advocacy is an important skill to develop when living with chronic pain. It means advocating for yourself in healthcare settings and communicating your needs effectively to providers. This can include advocating for pain management treatments that have worked for you, asking questions about treatment options, and expressing your concerns or needs regarding your care. Developing effective self-advocacy skills ensures you receive the care and support you need to manage your chronic pain effectively.

ANALOGY

Advocacy is like being the captain of your own ship. Just as a captain navigates their ship through rough waters, advocacy involves guiding yourself through the challenges of chronic pain. You are the one who knows your own needs and preferences, and you have the power to make decisions about your own care. Think of advocacy as being the captain of your own ship, as it allows you to take control of your life and navigate towards your desired destination with the necessary support and resources.

CONCLUSION

Building a support system is an essential part of coping with chronic pain. It can provide emotional, practical, and medical support, help you feel less isolated, and empower you to advocate for your needs. By finding the types of support you need and seeking out sources of support, you can improve your quality of life and build a more fulfilling and meaningful life despite chronic pain.

19. Overcoming the Stigma of Chronic Pain

Strategies for Addressing Misunderstanding and Bias in Society and Healthcare

INTRODUCTION

Millions of people worldwide are impacted by chronic pain, yet it is still widely misunderstood and stigmatised. Unlike acute pain, which is often a result of injury or illness and resolves when the underlying issue is treated, chronic pain is ongoing and can persist for months or years. As a result, it can affect every aspect of a person's life, from their ability to work and socialise to their mental and emotional well-being. Unfortunately, the stigma associated with chronic pain often makes individuals feel misunderstood, and even dismissed by society and healthcare providers.

This chapter explores the stigma associated with chronic pain and offers strategies for addressing it. By increasing awareness and understanding of this condition, I hope to help those with chronic pain feel supported, heard, and empowered. Through education, support, and advocacy, we can combat the negative perceptions surrounding chronic pain and enhance the well-being of individuals impacted by it.

THE STIGMA OF CHRONIC PAIN

Chronic pain is often invisible, meaning that others cannot

see the pain the individual is experiencing. This can lead to misunderstandings and scepticism from others, who may believe that the person with chronic pain is exaggerating or seeking attention. Additionally, the fact that chronic pain is often difficult to diagnose, and treat can add to the stigma associated with this condition.

The impact of this stigma can be far-reaching. Individuals with chronic pain may feel isolated and alone, exacerbating their pain and making it more challenging to manage. The stigma associated with chronic pain can also lead to a lack of understanding from healthcare providers, who may not take the condition seriously or may prescribe inadequate treatments.

STRATEGIES FOR ADDRESSING STIGMA

There are several strategies that individuals with chronic pain can use to address the stigma associated with this condition.

Firstly, education is an essential step in breaking down misconceptions and promoting a greater understanding of chronic pain. This can involve sharing personal experiences with chronic pain, discussing the science behind the condition, and advocating for better treatment options. In addition, education can help others understand the challenges faced by those with chronic pain, leading to increased empathy and support.

Secondly, seeking support from others experiencing similar challenges can be helpful in decreasing feelings of isolation and promoting a sense of belonging. Joining a chronic pain support group or online community can allow individuals to connect with other people who understand what they are going through and share coping strategies. This can help reduce the negative impact of stigma and enhance the quality of life for individuals with chronic pain.

Finally, advocating for better treatment options for chronic pain is crucial in reducing stigma and improving outcomes for individuals with this condition. This may involve working with your healthcare providers to find effective treatments or lobbying for policy changes prioritising the needs of those with chronic pain. In addition, you can play a vital role in increasing awareness and breaking down stigmas around chronic pain by sharing your experiences and highlighting the challenges faced due to this condition, ultimately leading to improved healthcare and social support for individuals with chronic pain.

STEPS TO IMPROVE STIGMA

Here are some more steps to address the stigma surrounding this condition:

- Utilise social media platforms to share personal stories and experiences with chronic pain. This can help raise awareness about the condition and reduce its associated stigma.
- Practice self-compassion and self-care. This involves being kind to oneself and taking time to engage in activities that promote physical and emotional well-being. In addition, self-compassion can help to counteract negative messages and stereotypes about individuals with chronic pain.

- Educate friends, family, and co-workers about chronic pain. This can involve providing resources and information about the condition, sharing personal stories, and dispelling myths and misconceptions.

- Seek professional mental health support to address the emotional toll of chronic pain and to develop coping strategies for dealing with stigma and social isolation.

- Get involved in advocacy efforts aimed at improving treatment options for chronic pain. This may include participating in research studies, lobbying for policy changes, or supporting organisations focusing on chronic pain advocacy and education.

By implementing these strategies, you can work towards reducing the stigma associated with this condition and promote greater understanding and support from your communities.

CONCLUSION

Chronic pain is indeed a complex condition that can be troublesome to handle. The stigma associated with chronic pain can exacerbate these challenges, leading to feelings of isolation and a lack of understanding from healthcare providers and others in society. By educating others, seeking support, and advocating for better treatment options, you can help address the stigma associated with this condition and improve your quality of life.

20. Managing Chronic Pain in the Workplace

Adapting Work Routines to Manage Pain

INTRODUCTION

Chronic pain can impact many areas of life, including work. For individuals with chronic pain, navigating the workplace can be challenging because of the pain, discomfort, and other symptoms which make it difficult to perform daily work activities. This chapter will discuss strategies for communicating with employers and colleagues about chronic pain, adapting work routines to manage pain, and maintaining productivity and job satisfaction despite chronic pain.

UNDERSTANDING CHRONIC PAIN AND THE WORKPLACE

Chronic pain can affect work in many ways, including reducing productivity, increasing absenteeism, and impacting job satisfaction. To effectively manage chronic pain, it is essential to understand its nature and how it can affect the workplace. Chronic pain can impact a person's ability to focus, concentrate, and complete tasks, which can lead to job dissatisfaction, increased stress, and a decrease in overall job performance.

COMMUNICATING WITH EMPLOYERS AND COLLEAGUES

Communication is vital when managing chronic pain in the workplace. Communicating with your employer and colleagues about your chronic pain and how it affects your work performance is essential. Educating your employer and colleagues about chronic pain and its impact on work can help them understand your situation and provide support. In addition, it is necessary to communicate any changes in work routines or accommodations needed to manage pain effectively.

ADAPTING WORK ROUTINES TO MANAGE PAIN

Managing chronic pain in the workplace often involves adapting work routines to accommodate pain symptoms. Strategies may include:

- Taking frequent breaks to stretch.
- Modifying workstations or equipment.
- Using assistive devices.
- Adjusting work schedules.

Finding ways to reduce physical stress and minimise pain triggers can also help manage pain in the workplace.

MAINTAINING PRODUCTIVITY AND JOB SATISFACTION

Managing chronic pain in the workplace can be challenging. Still, it is possible to maintain productivity and job satisfaction with the right strategies. For example, building a support system, setting realistic goals, and focusing on self-care can all help manage chronic pain and maintain a positive attitude at work. In addition, it is essential to prioritise rest and relaxation outside work to prevent burnout and effectively manage chronic pain symptoms.

EASY STEPS TO MANAGE PAIN AT WORK

I have detailed some additional strategies that can help manage chronic pain in the workplace below:

- Ergonomic setup: Ensure your workstation is ergonomically designed to minimize strain on your body. Adjust your chair height, desk height, and monitor position to maintain proper posture and reduce pain.

- Take regular breaks: Schedule short breaks throughout the day to give yourself time to stretch, move around, and relieve any built-up tension. Taking microbreaks every 30 minutes can help prevent pain from worsening.

- Modify your workspace: Make necessary modifications to your workspace to accommodate your needs. For example, use a cushioned chair, ergonomic keyboard, or footrest to reduce joint discomfort and pressure.

- Practice good posture: Maintain good posture when you are sitting or standing to alleviate strain on your body. Sit with your shoulders relaxed, back straight, and feet flat on the floor. Consider using lumbar support if needed.

- Use assistive devices: Utilize assistive devices such as wrist braces or speech recognition software to minimize pain and make tasks easier.

- Communicate with your employer: Openly communicate with your employer or supervisor about your chronic pain condition. Discuss any necessary accommodations or modifications to help you perform your job more effectively.

- Prioritize self-care: Engage in self-care activities outside work to manage your pain. This may include regular exercise, stretching, practising relaxation techniques, maintaining a healthy diet, and getting enough sleep.

- Break tasks into manageable chunks: Divide your tasks into smaller, more manageable portions to avoid prolonged periods of intense focus or physical strain. This approach can help prevent the exacerbation of pain and improve overall productivity.

- Utilize pain management techniques: Explore the pain management techniques discussed in the previous chapters to help you cope with pain while at work.

○ Seek support: Connect with colleagues, friends, or support groups who understand your situation. Sharing your experiences and challenges can provide emotional support and helpful tips for managing chronic pain in the workplace.

○ Using technology to manage pain: Many mobile apps and tools are available to help manage chronic pain in the workplace. For example, some apps provide reminders to take breaks and stretch. In contrast, others offer guided meditation or breathing exercises to help manage stress.

○ Developing a pain management plan: Working with a healthcare provider to develop a comprehensive pain management plan can help ensure you have effective strategies to manage pain while at work.

By implementing these additional strategies, you can better manage your symptoms in the workplace, improve job satisfaction, and maintain productivity.

CONCLUSION

Managing chronic pain in the workplace requires a multifaceted approach that includes communication with employers and colleagues, adapting work routines to accommodate pain symptoms, and maintaining productivity and job satisfaction. By taking proactive steps to manage chronic pain, you can continue to work productively, maintain a positive attitude, and achieve success in the workplace.

21. Advocacy and Empowerment

Becoming an Active Participant in Healthcare Decision-Making

INTRODUCTION

Dealing with chronic pain can be a challenging experience that can result in feelings of loneliness and detachment. However, it is vital to remember that you are not alone. In addition to seeking effective treatments for your pain, becoming an active participant in your healthcare and advocating for yourself and others living with chronic pain is essential. This chapter will provide the following:

- Strategies for becoming an informed and empowered patient.
- Communicating effectively with healthcare providers.
- Advocating for chronic pain research and funding.

BECOMING AN EMPOWERED PATIENT

Becoming an empowered patient involves taking an active role in your healthcare and working in partnership with your healthcare providers to manage your chronic pain. This includes educating yourself about your condition, understanding your treatment options, and advocating for your needs. It is essential to ask questions, express your concerns, and collaborate with your healthcare team. A holistic treatment plan that considers your physical, emotional, and social needs is crucial to effectively manage chronic pain.

EFFECTIVE COMMUNICATION WITH HEALTHCARE PROVIDERS

Effective communication with healthcare providers is essential for managing chronic pain. When discussing your pain with your healthcare provider, be specific about the location, intensity, and quality of your pain. Additionally, be sure to discuss any previous treatments or medications you have tried and any side effects you may have experienced. Finally, keeping a pain diary to track your pain levels and identify patterns or triggers can be helpful.

ADVOCATING FOR CHRONIC PAIN RESEARCH AND FUNDING

Advocacy for chronic pain research and funding is essential to raise awareness and support for individuals with chronic pain. This includes participating in advocacy efforts, sharing your story, and supporting organisations that advocate for chronic pain research and funding. You can also engage with policymakers and advocate for policies that improve access to effective pain management and support services.

CONCLUSION

Living with chronic pain can sometimes be a difficult and isolating experience. However, becoming an informed and empowered patient, communicating effectively with healthcare providers, and advocating for chronic pain research and funding can help manage your pain and improve your quality of life. By working together, we can raise awareness and support for individuals with chronic pain and enhance access to effective pain management and support services.

22. Pain and Relationships

Navigating Romantic and Familial Relationships When One Partner Has Chronic Pain

INTRODUCTION

Living with chronic pain can be challenging, not only for the person experiencing it but also for their loved ones. Chronic pain can impact all aspects of life, including relationships. The changes in daily routine, mood swings, and the inability to participate in activities that were once enjoyed can lead to frustration and stress in relationships. This chapter will explore the impact of chronic pain on romantic and familial relationships and provide strategies to navigate them.

THE IMPACT OF CHRONIC PAIN ON RELATIONSHIPS

Living with chronic pain can cause a ripple effect on relationships. Communication, intimacy, and support systems can be disrupted. Pain can create a power imbalance in a relationship, and the caregiver can feel overburdened. Often, the person with chronic pain may feel isolated and unsupported, leading to a feeling of guilt and worthlessness.

STRATEGIES TO HELP MANAGE RELATIONSHIPS

Patience and empathy:

It can be challenging for partners to understand chronic pain. Therefore, patience and empathy are critical when navigating relationships with chronic pain. In addition, both partners need to acknowledge that chronic pain can be unpredictable and may require extra support.

Communicating effectively:

Communication is critical to any relationship but especially crucial when one partner has chronic pain. Expressing feelings, needs, and limitations honestly and openly is essential. For example, if a romantic partner needs to cancel plans due to pain, it's vital to communicate that and not let the other partner assume that they are not interested. Communication can also help identify triggers and find ways to avoid them.

Understanding limitations:

Living with chronic pain often means accepting that there are limitations. Setting realistic expectations and goals is essential to avoid disappointment and feelings of failure. The person with chronic pain may have to adjust their schedule and activities, and the partner may need to be understanding and supportive.

Don't let chronic pain define the relationship:

While chronic pain can be a significant challenge, it's essential not to let it define the relationship. Instead, focusing on shared interests and hobbies, finding new activities to enjoy together, and celebrating milestones can help strengthen the bond between partners.

Maintaining intimacy:

Chronic pain can affect physical intimacy, but that doesn't mean it has to diminish the emotional bond between partners. Exploring other ways of intimacy, such as touching, hugging, and cuddling, can help maintain emotional closeness. It's important to communicate about physical intimacy and find ways to adapt to limitations caused by pain.

Building a support system:

A robust support system can help manage chronic pain and its impact on relationships. The partner can offer emotional support, but it's also essential to seek support from family, friends, or a support group. This can lessen the load on the partner and offer extra support to the individual dealing with chronic pain.

Seek professional help:

It may be helpful for the person with chronic pain and their partner to seek professional help, such as couples counselling. This can provide a safe space to communicate effectively and work through any issues that may arise.

Focus on self-care:

Both partners need to prioritise self-care. This includes getting enough rest, exercising regularly, eating healthily, and taking breaks when needed. In addition, by taking care of themselves, both partners can better support each other.

Be flexible:

Chronic pain can be unpredictable, and plans may need to change at the last minute. Being flexible and open to adjusting plans can help reduce stress and frustration.

CONCLUSION

Living with chronic pain can be challenging, but relationships can remain strong with communication, understanding, and support. It's important to remember that chronic pain not only affects the person with pain but also their loved ones. By working together and being open to adapting to new ways of living, relationships can thrive even in the face of chronic pain.

23. Supporting Your Loved Ones with Chronic Pain

Practical Tips for Family and Friends

INTRODUCTION

Dealing with chronic pain is like sailing on an unpredictable sea, where the waves of pain can rise and fall unexpectedly. Just like how a sailor needs a supportive crew to navigate through the rough waters, people with chronic pain need the support of their family and friends to cope with their condition. However, understanding how to provide that support can be difficult, especially when the pain is invisible. In this chapter, I will present some valuable advice to help you become a supportive ally for your loved ones who are dealing with chronic pain and assist them in managing their condition effectively.

ANALOGY

Picture yourself on a hiking excursion with the people you care about, and suddenly, one of them injures their leg. They are in excruciating pain, and the injury is not visible outside. You want to help them but don't know what to do. Should you carry them, or should they walk? Should you give them water, or should you find medical help? These questions may confuse you, but the truth is that you can help them by being a supportive companion, listening to their needs, and providing them with practical assistance. Similarly, dealing with chronic pain requires a supportive and understanding companion. You can be that person for your loved ones.

PRACTICAL TIPS

Here are some practical tips which can help.

- Listen actively: When your loved one talks to you about their pain, listen actively. This means really paying attention to what they're saying, asking questions to clarify anything unclear, and showing that you understand and empathize with what they're going through.

- Be patient: Chronic pain can be a frustrating and isolating experience for the person going through it. So, it's important to be patient with your loved one, even if they're not always able to perform the things they used to do or engage in recreations that they previously enjoyed.

- Help with daily tasks: Chronic pain can make it difficult for people to perform even simple daily tasks, like cooking or cleaning. Offering to help with these tasks helps your loved one and makes them feel more supported.

- Offer emotional support: Dealing with chronic pain can be an emotional rollercoaster. Your loved one may feel angry, frustrated, depressed, or anxious at different times. Offer emotional support by checking in regularly, providing a listening ear, and reminding your loved one that they're not alone.

- Be an advocate: Sometimes, people with chronic pain must fight to get the care they need. Be an advocate for your loved one, whether helping them find the right doctor or treatment or advocating for their needs with their employer or insurance company.

- Educate yourself: Learning more about chronic pain and its effects can help you be a better support system for your loved one. Many resources are available online or through support groups to help you understand what your loved one is going through and how best to support them.

- Offer to go with them to appointments: Chronic pain often requires medical attention, and appointments can be overwhelming. Offer to accompany your loved one to hospital appointments and take notes to help them remember what was discussed.

- Avoid giving unsolicited advice: It is advisable to refrain from giving unsolicited advice, despite the temptation to do so. Instead, trust that your loved one is doing their best to manage their pain and instead ask how you can support them.

- Encourage healthy habits: Encourage your loved one to maintain healthy habits such as eating well, exercising, and getting enough rest. These habits can help manage pain and improve overall well-being.
- Respect their limits: Chronic pain can be unpredictable, and your loved one may need to cancel plans or change their routine. Respect their limits and be understanding if plans need to be adjusted.

- Celebrate small victories: Living with chronic pain can be challenging, so celebrate your loved one's small victories. Whether completing a task or trying a new treatment, recognize their efforts and offer words of encouragement.

By following these practical tips, you can help your loved one feel more supported and understood as they navigate the challenges of chronic pain.

CONCLUSION

Supporting someone with chronic pain can be a daunting task. Still, it is essential to remember that your presence and support can make a significant difference in your loved one's life. By following these practical tips and adopting a compassionate and understanding approach, you can help your loved one manage their pain and improve their overall well-being. In addition, it is crucial to remember that chronic pain can be a long-term condition, and providing consistent and ongoing support can make a world of difference to your loved one's physical and emotional health.

About The Author

Dr Arul James M B B S, M D, F R C A, F F P M R C A

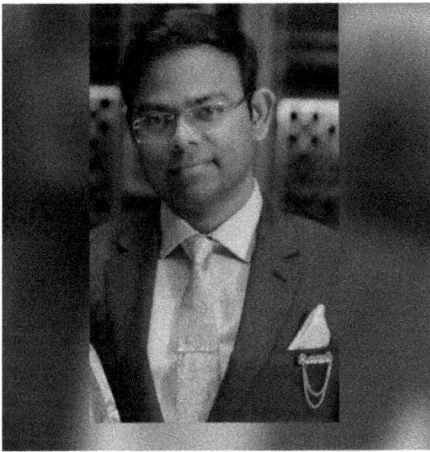

I am the Clinical Lead for Chronic Pain Medicine and Consultant in Chronic Pain Medicine and Anaesthetics at George Eliot Hospital NHS Trust in the West Midlands, United Kingdom. With a specialised focus on chronic pain, I possess a wealth of expertise in diagnosing and effectively treating a wide range of chronic pain conditions.

My foremost priority is providing patient-centred care. I collaborate closely with each individual to develop a personalised treatment plan tailored to their unique needs and goals.

Combining my deep understanding of chronic pain management with a compassionate approach, I strive to create a supportive and empathetic environment for my patients.

I am dedicated to delivering comprehensive and holistic care that encompasses various aspects of pain management, including medication management, interventional procedures, physical therapy, and lifestyle modifications. By addressing chronic pain's physical and emotional components, I aim to optimise your well-being and restore your ability to engage in daily activities and enjoy life to the fullest.

Feel free to share your feedback or get in touch:
https://www.aruljames.co.uk/